The Nine-Month Journey

The Nine-Month Journey

Sarah O'Connor

ABINGDON PRESS
Nashville

The Nine-Month Journey:
A Christian Mother's Reflections
on Pregnancy and Childbirth

Copyright © 1984 by Sarah O'Connor

Library of Congress Cataloging in Publication Data

O'CONNOR, SARAH, 1953-
The nine-month journey.
1. O'Connor, Sarah, 1953-   . 2. Pregnant women—United
States—Biography. 3. Pregnancy—Psychological aspects.
4. Pregnant women—Family relationships. 5. Christian life—
1960-   . I. Title. II. Title: 9-month journey.
RG525.026   1984   618.2 [B]   84-6485

ISBN 0-687-28017-6

Scripture quotations are from The Jerusalem Bible, copyright © 1966 by
Darton, Longman & Todd, Ltd. and Doubleday & Company, Inc. Used by
permission of the publisher.

"The Peace of Wild Things" by Wendell Berry appears on page 47,
copyright © 1968 by Wendell Berry. Reprinted from his volume *Openings*
by permission of Harcourt Brace Jovanovich, Inc.

MANUFACTURED BY THE PARTHENON PRESS AT
NASHVILLE, TENNESSEE, UNITED STATES OF AMERICA

To

Tom, Joseph, Brendan, and Peter

Contents

Introduction

When we were living in Boston, my husband and I met a middle-aged banker, a man happily married with three children. One day we happened to mention two friends of ours who were getting married. "Why such a desperate step?" was his response. I laughed, but his question was not entirely facetious.

Many people these days are ambivalent about marriage and, beyond that, about having children. In an article in a leading news magazine, women who did not want to have children were quoted. "I have hobbies and interests that I barely have time for now," one said. "Suddenly you're a mom and dad with a baby—it's no longer a lover relationship," said another. And, "We lead a full, fortunate life. I doubt if it would be any more rewarding with kids."

In a 1980 study of American families by two Harvard University sociologists *(The Nation's Families: 1960-1990)*, Professors Mary Jo Bane and George Masnick reported that by 1990, nearly two-thirds of the households in the United States will be childless. By 1990 the traditional nuclear family will no longer be the American norm. Other factors will accelerate this movement. Divorce rates probably will continue to climb. More people will choose to lead single lives. And women will continue to choose careers other than mothering and homemaking. Husband-wife households with only one partner working outside the home will drop to 14 percent by 1990, as compared to 43 percent in 1960.

Most households without children will be so by choice. Many women will not want to interrupt their careers, and many couples will want or need a double income. Some couples will fear the changes children will bring in their lives together, while others will choose not to have children because of fears about overpopulation or the feeling that the world is a bad place with an uncertain future. Why bring children into it? In light of all that is involved, "Why such a desperate step?" becomes a legitimate question.

For that reason I decided to record some of my thoughts and experiences as I began a new phase in my life—motherhood. I had questions and worries like all women, but I have written this book in the hope that my experiences will help other women feel less alone when they decide to have children and encourage those who might want children but who feel, as I did, anxious about the consequences.

Prelude (June to July)

June 29. Rain for three days and nights. Last night I woke up to the sound of thunder and flashes of lightning. Now the rain has stopped, but it is damp and humid. I can hear the cars swishing by and a couple of birds whistling. How pleasant to sit here on our bed with no other sounds but those of the outdoors. Outside my window, drops of water bounce off mini-trampolines as they hit the surface of the leaves.

July 2. I was tired at work today. My body felt like a heavy weight. This rainy and humid weather makes me want to stay in bed in the morning.

July 4. Fourth of July. We went to Tom's sister's house for a cookout and to watch the parade. Most of the town was in the parade. Everyone seemed happy and filled with patriotic energy, but I felt tired and vaguely depressed.

July 5. Tonight we dropped by a Greek restaurant on Main Street. It brought back memories of six weeks I spent in Greece in the summer of 1967 with a high school group. I remember expecting that in a foreign country I would be a different person—less awkward and more sophisticated. I discovered that I was the same person in Greece as in America. Only the place changed. I still got bored, made mistakes, reacted negatively. There was no escape from myself. In fact, being in a foreign country made me more aware of myself as an individual. I stood out from the culture around me, isolated and vulnerable.

The few times when I did not feel like a tourist and a stranger stand out: In a country restaurant beside a noisy waterfall we picked cherries and ate freshly baked bread along with a party of Greek travelers. Somehow I felt that I was part of the group. Why? A few days later we stopped at a little cafe along a dusty road. Several men were drinking coffee at the tables. After we had lemonade, the men were easily cajoled into showing us Greek dances. In the back room, three men circled and turned to the sometimes melancholy, sometimes wildly exuberant music. Then all fifteen of us joined in. We had been accepted. The rest of the hot afternoon passed quickly, sightseeing forgotten.

Tomorrow is a big day. We will see what it brings.

July 6. I was right. Today is a big day. I am pregnant. I don't know what to think. I was expecting the news, but at the same time, part of me thought it would never happen. I know pregnancy will change everything, but perhaps I should think of it as a journey to a foreign country. In eight months I will be in another country, but I will still be the same person. Tom will be the same person. And after we've been there for a time, it will no longer be a foreign country; it will be home.

I hadn't told Tom I might be pregnant because I have thought so before and have been wrong. I had the test this morning and called about the results in the afternoon. When I called, the woman on the other end of the line said, "Would there be any problem if the results were positive?" —a question no one would have asked our mothers. What would she have said if I had answered yes? How many of the babies of women who answer yes actually see this world?

I told her there would be no problem, and she replied, "In that case, the test is positive." When she said that, I lost touch with reality for a moment. Was she talking to me? Was it true? Hadn't there been a slight tremor in the floor when she made her announcement? Yet everything around me looked normal, as if nothing had happened.

Tom and I went out for dinner after work. I had been

12

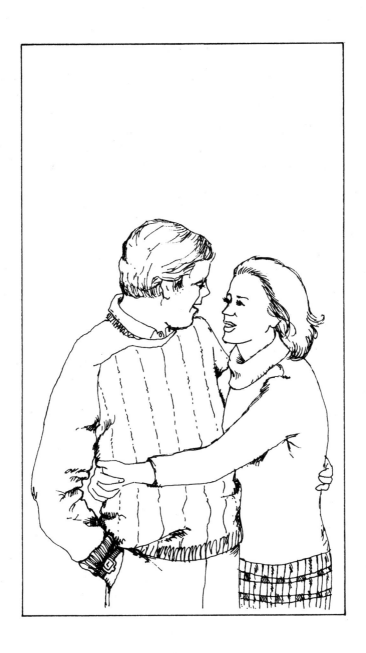

trying to think of a way of telling him without simply blurting it out. We talked about friends and the day's events for awhile. Then I said, "I have some news for you." He casually asked what. "*Big* news," I said. Then he guessed what the news was, got excited, and decided that he needed a glass of wine. We went home half-dazed with pleasure and half-frightened by our knowledge that our lives were about to change irrevocably.

A New Life (July to November)

July 8.   The idea of being pregnant has sunk in a little more. It seems a miracle that I (or anyone) could ever get pregnant. So much has to go right for an egg to be fertilized. In the book *A Child Is Born*, Lennart Nilsson says:

> Actually, it is rather strange that we exist at all. One single ovum, small as the point of a pin, is released into the abdominal cavity every fourth week. What if it were to get lost and fail to enter the Fallopian tube, where the sperm have only hours to find it among all folds and recesses?

Reading that passage makes me think about what actually occurred to allow this baby to begin forming inside me.

It really started a long time ago. I, like every woman, was born with a million or two primordial egg cells already formed within me. Only one ripens a month—only about four hundred total during my fertile years.

So, first one of these egg cells ripens and rises to the surface of the ovary encased in a sac called the follicle. When the egg is ready, the sac breaks open, releasing it into the abdominal cavity. The sac then releases hormones to stop the ripening of any other eggs, to signal the Fallopian tubes to move the egg on toward the uterus, and to tell the uterus to prepare itself for the fertilized egg.

In order for the egg to be fertilized, sometime just before or while the egg moves toward the uterus, sperm has to pass through the mucous membrane of the cervix. During most of the menstrual cycle, the mucous membrane is so thick that the sperm cannot penetrate it, but during the fertile part of the cycle, the mucous becomes thin and clear, so that the sperm can easily move through. After the sperm pass through the cervix, they swim up into the Fallopian tubes

15

and arrive at just the right time in the journey of the ovum (egg) in order to fertilize it.

When the ovum is released, it is surrounded by a cluster of follicle cells. The Fallopian tube secretions wash these away, leaving only a gelatinous coating. The sperm has to penetrate that coating and then penetrate the ovum's surrounding thin cell membrane. Once inside, the sperm dissolves, releasing its genetic material. At the same time the cell's membrane changes to prevent other sperm from entering.

After fertilization, there are still many chances for the egg to be lost. It must continue its precarious journey down the Fallopian tube and become properly embedded in the uterine wall. Then it must receive adequate nourishment in order to remain there. (In spite of the seemingly common-place nature of pregnancy, about 17 percent of otherwise normal American couples have fertility problems, which illustrates the hazards involved.)

All things considered, I am awestruck that I am here. I am awestruck that such a complex and beautiful process could be happening inside me. I wonder why this particular egg and sperm came together out of the millions of other possible combinations. The world will be changed in a particular way, whether large or small, because of the unique personality of this still tiny fragment of life.

So far this tiny being has not put so much as a dent in my routine. I go to work every day, clean the house, cook meals. I have not felt sick or especially hungry. The awareness is with me, though, that I am not alone.

July 14. It is extremely humid and has been for days. The air is dead. Mushrooms are springing up in neighboring yards because of the dampness. The humidity increases my lassitude.

July 21. I am feeling sick now. Even before I get out of bed in the morning, I experience nausea. The best solution seems to be to throw myself into activities that take my mind off of pregnancy.

I find myself thinking about having a baby as something entirely separate from my past life. Actually, however, the baby will be a natural continuation of my life with Tom and a way for our marriage to continue to grow and branch out.

Children affirm that we remain participants in the cycles of the earth: birth, life, death, rebirth. We are all part of these cycles, no matter how much we deny them or ignore them. "Yes," I say to life. "Yes, I do want to be part of you."

July 22. I have sometimes experienced depression and lack of hope, which have at their root the failure to assent to life, its trials as well as its joys. I said, "Yes, I want to be part of life" but affirmation is not a one-time matter. That yes, which is actually a yes to God and what he intends for me, must be repeated continuously. It is a matter of will as well as faith. In *No Man Is an Island*, Thomas Merton says, "The modern world is beginning to discover, more and more, that the quality and vitality of a man's life depend on his own secret will to go on living."

The will to go on does not appear to be related to objective situations. Some people crumble under the smallest amount of adversity. Others retain their will to live despite conditions as difficult as prison camp and physical torture. Letting go of the will to live, refusing to say yes to life, is accepting a certain degree of death in life. Death does not have to come suddenly. It can gradually seep into our being so that we hardly notice its presence.

August 16. Tom is out of town for a few days. I miss him, but it is good to be here in peace and quiet, listening to the night sounds.

17

I worry that I am going to have to get used to doing without these quiet times after the baby comes. I will have to be able to carry my peace within me then, since I will be unable to draw it from frequent periods of solitude. Quiet does not always bring peace, anyway. I can be in a totally quiet place and still be restless and anxious. Conversely, I can be in the midst of confusion and noise but have peace. Peace is a gift from God. Perhaps having a baby will bring a new and deeper peace than what I now experience.

I am still feeling sick off and on, even with the medication the doctor prescribed. Everyone says three months is the turning point, though. That means two more weeks. My skirts are tight in the waist. I get tired and sometimes feel depressed, but for the most part I am happy. My father told me, "You have that 'I have a secret' look in your eyes." It's true. I carry around the knowledge of being pregnant constantly. Almost every hour a new aspect of that knowledge presents itself to me, but the most basic fact is that I am on a journey into the unknown. That fact underlies all my fears and hopes, and it demands faith, not knowledge. I remember how the Lord provided for us when we faced other challenges, and I believe that he will provide just as generously in the future.

August 18. The sky has become overcast, and the air is heavy. Smells hang in the air instead of being blown away. It is already mid-August.

I tried taking a nap this afternoon. Result: one headache. I do not think I am a napper.

Today I went running. I am used to running two or three miles a day. I ran only one mile, but it felt great. No one can tell I am pregnant yet, so I do not feel self-conscious. The test will come when I begin to show. Perhaps I will run in the evening then. I saw an ad a few days ago for a maternity jogging suit. What next?

I think I can feel my uterus slightly. It is a hard place in my lower abdomen. The baby is almost three inches long now. In two more weeks I will be three months pregnant. It is hard to believe. In two more weeks the baby will officially become a fetus rather than an embryo.

September 18. I am into my fourth month now, and that is all I can think about. The thought constantly distracts me when I talk to other people. How will we arrange the furniture in the study to make it into a baby's room? When will I feel the baby move? Am I gaining too much weight? Who will coach me in labor? What will life be like after the baby is born? Will it be a boy or a girl? I can be thinking about politics or the weather or what to have for dinner when the realization suddenly strikes me anew that I, Sarah O'Connor, am pregnant. I will have a baby. This is happening to me.

Why is it so hard for me to believe I am pregnant? If I have a choice, I usually choose to be an observer in a situation rather than an actor. Often I want to be invisible, not noticed. Why is it threatening to be noticed? There are days when all relationships seem artificial. My words, their words, seem like games played for amusement or to pass the time. After playing, everyone leaves, satisfied they have performed well. I am uncomfortable allowing people into the deeper levels of my life. Is this selfish? Am I becoming self-absorbed, or am I being gradually possessed by the child that my body is creating?

I want to pray for freedom from fears about the future, freedom from feeling defeated in relationships and in projects before I've even begun them. I want more hope and self-confidence.

19

It is winter already. The first snow has fallen and the trees are bare. The darkness comes early. It is a season of reflection.

November 11. I am waiting for the parts of my life to converge. This time before the baby comes should be a period for reflection and taking stock. Caring for my inner life is like caring for a plant. Clip back the trailing, unproductive ends, and new shoots flourish around the roots. I am cutting back on some of my unnecessary activities, waiting for a fuller inner life to emerge.

November 18. I asked myself Sunday whether there was anything preventing me from coming closer to God, and I felt that he brought two things to mind. First, I acknowledge his protection in the past, but I lack confidence in the future. I fail in my faith that God will continue to be with us and do good things for us. Second, I realize that I have not been accepting the present. I have been unconsciously dissatisfied with my friends, my job, with Tom—even with the fact that I am pregnant. I repented because I know God's loving nature and have experienced his love. Since then I have felt great peace and a sense of looking forward to the future. I am in God's hands, part of his providential design. All of my decisions are touched by his love so that they are his as well as mine.

Quite indifferent to these thoughts, the baby has been kicking happily at my stomach for a couple of months now. No worries about the future there!

Tom is in New Jersey today. This pregnancy has been a good time for us. I experience him caring for me and being concerned about me, and I see how much I need him. He is a source of strength. Interdependence is better than independence.

November 19.

> The spinning that will not stop.
>> a knot that tightens
>> as the days tighten toward winter.
>
> Falling and sliding—
>> where will it end?
>
> Father, what place is this
>> where the light is blurred ahead
>> and the past falls behind?

I envy those with their lives firmly under control. Such persons must be wholly creative, and I feel dismay at my own situation. I wonder if I will ever find my place. This is a question that can only be answered through faith in God's providence.

January

January 5.   Today I am overcome with the finality of what Tom and I have done and fearful of all the changes it will bring. The Christmas holidays were so busy that I did not have time to think about the baby. We visited my parents in Washington and had a joyful reunion. My brothers are excited over the prospect of becoming uncles, but most of the time was spent reminiscing.

Now I must think about getting things ready here at home. We need a crib. The furniture in the study has to be rearranged. And I want to re-cover the cushions on the rocking chair. The baby is real and will be here soon.

Strangely enough, my thoughts about having a baby have been intertwined with thoughts about death. Two years ago, after the death of the son of a friend, I began to think about death as something real for the first time and to be afraid of it. I found myself going through the normal events in my life and suddenly being struck with the thought that I was going to die someday. I even had nightmares about dying. The fear of death kept surfacing no matter what I was doing.

The example of Jesus helped me to accept death. He recognized death and walked toward it calmly. He did not want to die, even though he knew he would rise again, but he accepted the will of his Father and went with courage. Better to stand before an enemy and fight than to flee. I know that when the time comes I will not go through death alone, because God's strength will be with me.

When I first learned that I was pregnant, I could not picture myself after having a child, as though I would be different or, in a sense, dead afterwards. I thought of all the things I should do before having a child, much like a person making a will. It is odd that birth should bring thoughts of death. As I walked to the car the other day, I was struck with the thought, "I am going to have a baby," and I noticed that it came just the way my thoughts that I would die someday used to come.

January 6. Having a first child does seem like a kind of death. Having a child is an entry into the unknown. The *before* is known, but not the *after*. It is like being able to see down a corridor to a door but not knowing what is behind that door. All I have heard is reports (not always positive) about what others found there. How different will life be after this child? How will my relationship with Tom be affected? Will I be happy or will I feel trapped? Will I become, simply, a mother? Will people stop relating to me as a person?

I now know that there are many small deaths in life, and some not so small. Even to live a day-to-day existence demands courage. Jesus is the model. Keeping our eyes on him, we can walk out of those deaths into new life.

Getting married was a small death to an old way of life, an embracing of a certain unknown, an act of faith in Tom and in God. Having a child is another. There is no going back. It is a time to take courage and to believe that we do not go into any unknown alone.

Today I looked at the calendar and counted the weeks since I became pregnant. I have seven and a half weeks to go. That means only one more month to prepare, since the baby may come early. There is so much to do. Yet the tailor's shop where I work is so busy that I would feel guilty about quitting earlier than I had planned.

Until recently it was not hard to keep working. I was rarely tired the first three months. In these last three months, however, I have gone through periods of being physically exhausted. I have even succumbed to a couple of naps. In spite of feeling tired, I enjoy my work. On the other

23

hand, I need to have time to think about this change in my life and to prepare a room for the baby. The two will go hand in hand. Getting a place ready for the baby is a way of preparing myself, and I know I will feel more peaceful once we have a crib and changing table set up. The nesting instinct, some people call it.

I am now completely and very obviously pregnant. Tom keeps telling me that I have never looked better, but I worry that I am putting on too much weight. Well, in a month and a half I will go back to jogging. Right now I lack the energy.

January 7. In the eighth month of pregnancy the baby is supposed to weigh five and one-quarter pounds and be eighteen inches long. That will be in two more weeks. I walked to work today, and although I was sitting much of the day, when I walked home my lower abdomen ached. I am feeling heavy. The ligaments attached to the uterus must be under tremendous strain.

I will not work full time past this week. I do not want to be caught in the position of a friend who thought she would have three weeks to prepare after she stopped working and then had her baby five weeks early.

It is bitterly cold outside. I am happy to be curled at the end of the couch with my pen and paper and books. Nothing seems more natural to me than sitting with a good book. When I was younger, my sister constantly tried to persuade me to go outside with her to play. Whenever I agreed, it was with reluctance. My real world lay between the covers of a book. The outside world was not as interesting. I was happiest when left alone for hours. Sometimes, after long periods engrossed in a book, I began to lose touch with reality. The outside world would become strange, and the world in my book would seem the real one.

I think that my enjoyment of a meditative, slow-paced

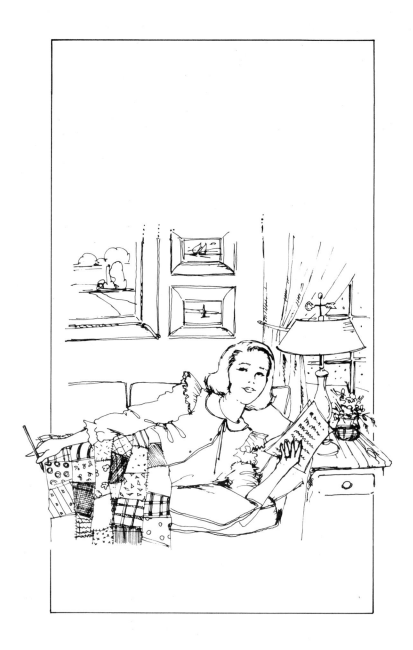

existence will be a benefit when I am staying at home. I know that much of my attention will be demanded by my baby, but I hope there will also be time for reading, thinking, and writing. How realistic is this? I do not know . . . another of those unknowns.

One of the hardest things about being at home is being self-motivated. No one is around to pat me on the back for a good job or to tell me to get moving if the job is not going well. Chores are chores, and the glamour of being at home wears off fast. I hope to get used to it during the next month when I will not be working.

The problem of motivation is not new to me. Anyone who writes faces it. Like many other writers I have written articles without knowing if they would be published. I have persisted without encouragement. I know the experience of thinking of important things that need doing as soon as I have hit the first typewriter key. Writing is an acid test for self-motivation, and I have failed it many times. The biggest obstacle to overcome has been myself. There is a voice inside every writer that shouts, "It's no good" as soon as two or three sentences have appeared on a fresh sheet of typing paper.

I would not be surprised if that voice liked to say the same sort of thing to mothers: "You're doing a lousy job!" The internal critic can speak to anyone, but people who work alone are particularly subject to it. Like writing, being a housewife and mother must be a lonely and a bitterly discouraging job at times.

January 8. It is becoming common for couples to decide not to have children. When Tom and I were considering parenthood, part of me wanted a child and part of me resisted the idea. What woman does not wonder about her ability to be a mother, wonder whether she will like it or not, wonder how it will affect her life? It is much easier to cling to the status quo than to take risks, but what is life without risks?

Bad news in the newspapers! Russians in Afghanistan. The Pope fears a nuclear buildup by the super powers. War is on everyone's mind but no one mentions the word. Our energy supplies are running out. Overpopulation. Famine.

How can anyone bring a child into this world? Besides fears about my own ability to mother, I have fears about the future of the world. Will there be a decent world by the time my baby has become an adult? I answer that question for myself by faith in God. I have faith that God will care not only for me but for my child as well.

Most parents would like to protect their children from all the hardships of life but that is impossible. Instead we need to give our children the tools to meet difficult situations. The most important of those tools is faith. Christians know that their children are born not only for this world but also for the eternal kingdom of God.

I have found life to be good. Even when it is hard, life is worth living. I want to pass that life on. I will struggle to overcome obstacles in my life, to swim among the waves, to retain my hope. My child may eventually decide life is not a good thing, but I will not have decided that for my child by refusing it a chance to live. I hope my child will come to the conclusion I have—that life is a supreme privilege.

I was so sore around my lower abdomen last night that I could hardly walk. Today I feel better. Next time I go to the doctor I will ask about how to reduce the discomfort.

January 9. Last night I felt overwhelmed again by the idea of having a baby. So much needs to be done. I spent the morning with mothers with young babies and after dinner helped a couple who had just moved into a new apartment.

They had two children. Being around all those children did not make me want one. I expect to feel differently, though, when it is my own.

Lately I have been moody. I get angry easily. If Tom does not help me, I get mad. I overreact to situations. Probably I am overtired.

Tonight is our Lamaze class. That is another factor in my moodiness. Too much thinking about babies. Right now we need a good movie more than a Lamaze class.

Tom and I have started praying together in the mornings. We are both used to taking time in the mornings for solitary prayer, but we have not spent much time praying together. It is a good way to start the day and gives us a sense of togetherness. We begin by thanking God for being with us and working in our lives. Then we read a psalm and a passage from the New Testament. Then we pray some more, bringing in our plans for the day.

We also take time once a week to talk. We like to go out for dessert or just a cup of coffee together during that time. We do not always have a great deal to discuss, but the custom helps keep lines of communication open. I need a lot of Tom's love now.

For some time I have been doing exercises from Elisabeth Bing's book, *Moving Through Pregnancy*. Exercises make a big difference in how I feel. I do not get leg cramps or feel stiff when I do them regularly. Some of the book's exercises are the same ones we are taught in the Lamaze class. They are supposed to help make the delivery easier by toning up the abdominal muscles. They are also supposed to reduce soreness after delivery and to make it easier to regain some sort of a figure.

One more day of work! How nice. This will be the first time in five years I have not been working.

January 12.   When I first got married, I used to wonder what it would mean to be a wife, a married woman. The adjustment was not easy but in time it came. Everything worked together to produce gradual answers to my question.

I suppose being a mother is similar. I wonder what it is, whether I can do it and whether I will like it. Being a mother does not seem like "me," but time and trial and error will probably answer my questions.

Several days ago we went to a couple's house for dinner. The wife related her dream about giving birth. In her dream she had the baby, but then left it in a bedroom and forgot it for three weeks. When she remembered the baby, it was fine but very hungry. She could not remember its name.

I have had similar dreams. These dreams must come from a fear of inadequacy in a new role (will I do everything right?) and an ambivalence toward the being who will change so much in my life. Most women probably experience these feelings, even if only subconsciously.

Taking on the role of mother is unlike marriage in that I won't be leaving behind a previous role to assume a new one. The roles of wife and lover are already established, and the role of mother is added to them. I will have to wait until after the baby comes to know how that role modifies the others.

Tom and I went to another Lamaze class. I enjoyed it more than the first one. The couples were more relaxed with one another. The class made me feel excited about the approaching labor.

The day after the Lamaze class, I went to see the doctor. I had written down questions to ask him but was too embarrassed to pull out my notebook when I reached the office. Consequently, I forgot to ask what to take for heartburn.

The doctor reminded me that I should not expect the baby

29

in February (a letdown after the Lamaze class). Also, I saw I had gained five more pounds. That makes twenty-five pounds already and I probably have over a month and a half left. Horrors! I have to watch my carbohydrates. That is hard because I love bread and sweets. Today, after firm resolves otherwise, I ate the icing off a piece of cake. It was delicious!

Yes, a long time to go yet. I should take a vacation. Florida? Swim, sunbathe, forget babies for a while. I *am* dreaming now.

At the Lamaze class we were told the necessity of picking a focal point to concentrate on during labor. That made me think about my need for a focal point in life, something which is the center of my life and gives it meaning. For some people the focal point is a job, children, or a car. As a Christian, I believe that focal point should be Jesus. When all other things pass away, he will remain. "I am the Way, the Truth and the Life," he said. He is the way through difficulties, the way to the kingdom of God, the truth in the universe where all truth seems relative, and the life that will never die. He gives meaning to the different roles we pass through.

January 14.   I am becoming convinced that it is possible to read too much about birth. The same thing is true of books on raising children—every book offers different advice. It is certainly good to be informed, but I tend to read several books on a given subject and end up overwhelmed by the conflicting information. Then I have to call a halt and return for a day or two to my mystery novels or do some cooking—anything to make life less confusing. Some books on birth try so hard to set my mind at ease that they end up convincing me that there must be something to worry about.

Today I had a visit with the obstetrical nurse. She answered some questions about how the delivery would go—very pleasant but routine. How can I or anyone become anything but another face to nurses and doctors? Do they only treat dying patients with consideration? Do they *even* treat dying patients with consideration?

I go to a clinic in which four doctors are in a joint practice. I learned today what some of their policies are regarding delivery. They do preps (shaving of pubic hair) and episiotomies for first deliveries. They will not allow labor-room deliveries for first babies, and they use i.v.'s in the delivery room. All of these practices are ones on which medical opinion varies. My doctors take a traditional approach. One newer practice they allow is a dimming of lights after the baby is born. I asked about this because I had read that strong lights in the delivery room can bother a newborn baby's eyes.

I like the doctor I have. She is young and has had two babies of her own. There is only a 25 percent chance of getting her for the delivery, though. The four doctors rotate being on call.

It is easy during this time to be too introspective. My body is like a workshop I am continually observing, acutely aware of the smallest changes. This physical self-consciousness lends itself to an emotional self-consciousness. I can be talking with friends and suddenly realize I have not been listening to what they are saying. I have been off daydreaming. People encourage my inward focus by repeatedly asking me how I am feeling. The obvious solution is to take the focus off myself, to look for ways of serving others.

January 15. Nights have a become a series of trips to the bathroom and tossing to find a comfortable position. I have begun sleeping on my side with a pillow between my legs.

This morning for exercise I walked over to a shopping center about half a mile away. The temperature was 30 degrees, but it felt invigorating. Instead of putting my hat on, I let the wind blow past my ears and chill my face. When I left I was feeling tired and ill, but as I walked I began feeling better. There is a balance between too much rest and too little. Too much rest makes my joints ache when I stand up, too little makes me irritable.

Holiness—what does it have to do with me, I've been wondering. Is my life supposed to be holy?

Paul, in his first letter to the Thessalonians, says, "What God wants is for you all to be holy" (4:3). The answer is yes, then. But what does that mean? Holiness connotes something removed from ordinary life, above it. I think of a state too high and awesome for the average person to attain. The word brings to mind scenes of Moses before the burning bush, St. Francis being raised off the ground during prayer, the mystical writings of Saint John of the Cross, etc.

I believe those things happened, and I believe we can experience moments of ecstasy or see visions, but I do not believe that miracles are the criteria for determining holiness.

Looking through the Bible at the various references to holiness, I see that God is spoken of as the Holy One. Being holy is being like God, taking on his nature. That is possible, not through our own efforts, but through the action of Jesus in dying and rising so that our sins can be forgiven and we can receive the Holy Spirit, God living in us. Holiness can only come through faith in the Son of God. Faith is not only mental assent, it is trust and obedience as well.

God created us and gives us the privilege of living in union with him. It is a privilege because of the great love he has for us. It is a chance to be loved and to love in return. The call to holiness is God's initiative. Our part is to respond.

The response is day-by-day, moment-by-moment. The smallest events in life can be opportunities for growing in holiness. While changing a diaper or hoeing the garden we can be turning to God. "And we, with our unveiled faces reflecting like mirrors the brightness of the Lord, all grow brighter and brighter as we are turned into the image that we reflect; this is the work of the Lord who is Spirit" (2 Cor. 3:18). Holiness comes down to the small choices we make and the way most of us live out our normal and, at times, mundane lives.

It is faith in Christ that gives meaning to existence. The most exciting job can be meaningless without faith. Likewise, the most routine work can have meaning because of our faith.

Women today, myself included, are afraid of the routine of caring for children, home, and husband. Indeed, it is the mundane and routine that threaten to crush the life out of us. But *that* is the challenge. If we cannot find God in our ordinary lives, where can we find him? He cannot be available only to those people who go off to another country to become missionaries or to those who live solitary lives of prayer and contemplation.

Women at home wonder if their lives are significant. What is produced is so intangible. But God does not measure our worth by dazzling public achievements. We were all created by God, and we each have intrinsic worth. We receive our identity from being sons and daughters of God. The work we do is an expression of that identity, so whether we are working at home or at a job, or both, we have equal value in God's eyes.

January 16. Another concern for me is what it will be

33

like to be on my own with children to take care of. I am afraid of nothingness, of aloneness, but the answer is not to lose myself among other people. Down deep the fear and aloneness will remain. The answer is to face it and accept it in the knowledge that it is a God-given challenge.

I know, no matter what it will be like, that God will be in the midst of it, at the very heart of it, and that it will be a job that calls forth love. I remind myself that the worst thing in the world is to be separated from God. As Paul says in Romans 8, "Nothing therefore can come between us and the love of Christ, even if we are troubled or worried, or being persecuted, or lacking food or clothes, or being threatened or even attacked. As scripture promised: 'For your sake we are being massacred daily and reckoned as sheep for the slaughter,' These are the trials through which we triumph, by the power of him who loved us" (35-37).

Another passage in scripture that speaks to me now is: "Fear is driven out by perfect love" (I John 4:18). My fears about the future indicate that I have not come to know the love of God perfectly. I have not come to the point of perfect trust in him. I repent when I begin to feel anxious about the future. It is not that I think all lack of faith is a matter for repentance. But for me now, lack of faith is a turning away from what I know about the nature of God. I have seen him working in my life so frequently that I have become responsible for my attitude. For me, it is a betrayal of God not to trust him. It is saying that I do not believe his nature is loving in spite of his many gifts to me. It is giving in to self-pity or to momentary doubts when I should stand firm in the truth. I have to keep up my part of the relationship.

I spoke to a friend about feeling obsessed with the thought of the baby coming. She said my attitude was natural. The same thing had happened to her during the last two months before her baby was born. She called my attitude "tunnel vision."

Sleeping is still not comfortable. I get up at least four times to go to the bathroom, and my mind keeps turning things over.

Tom uses the car for work, so I have become used to going places on foot. Yet even a twenty-minute walk seems long now. That is how long it took me to walk to a friend's house this morning. My body adjusted to the weight of the baby after a while.

While I was walking I noticed how few colors and sounds there are in the winter. Color is important to human beings. Lack of color and sound makes life seem dreary. There were no birds singing. Even the sounds of cars were muffled in the cold, damp air. Spring is such a joy when it comes. It is a bombardment of the senses after a long deprivation. I am certain much of the depression people experience in the winter is caused by sensory deprivation, even though they are unaware of what they are missing.

January 18. This pregnancy is going to go on forever! The due date is still so far away. At least another month and a half. I ran into someone today who said the last month is the longest of your life. Very reassuring.

I am frustrated at every turn in trying to get ready. I have looked for a nightgown that buttons down the front and is feminine. Finally I bought something, but not at all what I had in mind. Remembering the episode, I have to laugh. I was in the dressing room of a fancy lingerie shop. What with the small size of the room and the large size of my stomach, I could hardly turn around. An older woman was helping me, bringing one nightgown after another. I spent a long time deciding. Finally I narrowed the choice to two but agonized further before making my purchase. I am sure the saleswoman could not understand my anxiety. Or maybe she remembered. As I looked in the mirror I tried to picture how each nightgown would look without the stomach. The nightgown had to make me look pretty and desirable. It had to be a kind of celebration. I wanted to feel like a woman again. A tall order—no wonder I had such a hard time picking it out.

Today my mother called to say she would come as soon as I was out of the hospital. I had planned to ask her to come a week later, but it will be better to have her here right away. It will be humbling to have her witness all my mistakes. This is a vulnerable time, but I am resigned to it. I can't always present a flawless image.

January 20. Tom and I have decided that my friend Rebecca will be my labor coach. (I have been taking Lamaze classes to learn breathing techniques to help me relax and stay in control during labor. People using the method choose a "coach" to be with them during labor to encourage them and coach them on their breathing.) Having had three babies herself, Rebecca will understand better than Tom could what I am going through. Tom will still be there the whole time. He will talk to the doctors and nurses, come in and out of the labor room, and go into the delivery room with me.

While I was practicing breathing techniques with Rebecca, I felt embarrassed to be in the position of needing to be taken care of. When I was about five years old, I thought it would be fun to break an arm or leg because of all the attention I would get. Once during a visit to my grandmother I hurt my foot. Being a nurse, she bandaged it, put me in a chair, and declared me a temporary invalid. To my surprise I hated being cared for. I did not like being helpless and the more considerate she became, the more unhappy I felt. As soon as I could, I left the chair and removed the bandage.

Everyone likes to feel self-sufficient, but the desire to be independent is one of the attitudes that keeps us from being close to God and to one another. We think we do not need him, that it is more admirable to succeed on our own.

Jesus told his disciples to leave everything to follow him but not because they were wealthy or because they owned the wrong kind of possessions. No, Jesus wanted their hearts to be empty of anything that separated them from him in order to show them that only God could fill their deepest need. They had to put themselves entirely in God's hands to find that out.

It is hard to concentrate when I try to pray. My mind keeps wandering to what I need to do to prepare for the baby. Yet I know the interior preparation is even more important than the exterior. How can I quiet my mind and heart to pray? It must become harder as more children come and there is ever more to be done. Women have probably been trying to solve this problem for centuries.

One advantage in being at home is that I will be able to control my environment. I can make my home conducive to a relationship with God. Seeing something beautiful can make me feel closer to God. That raises the difficult question of what is beautiful and why beauty has any relation to God. Much of what anyone considers beautiful is predetermined by childhood experiences, parental attitudes, the chance influences of what one is exposed to in architecture, social status, geography, climate, and the like. Added to these influences is the influence of education: art classes, music classes, trips to museums or to foreign countries. These influences, however, are not decisive. They do not create a sense of beauty. Rather, they make us aware of our own interior sense of proportion, space, color, and harmony. I believe these interior perceptions are summed up in our sense of the truth of what we see. Does what we see correspond with our intuitive sense of beauty? The interior perceptions are innate, God-given. They are also the foundations upon which the universe was created. I think they reflect the nature of the Creator.

The Japanese weave beauty into the fabric of their lives. Most Japanese families have a small garden, no matter how tiny their homes are. I would like to try to find ways to bring more beauty into our home. In Philippians 4:8 Paul writes, "Finally, brothers, fill your minds with everything that is true, everything that is noble, everything that is good and pure, everything that we love and honor, and everything that can be thought virtuous or worthy of praise." One way to raise our minds to those things is to surround ourselves with beautiful things. Not necessarily expensive, these beautiful things can be anything from a seashell to a vase of fresh flowers to a lovely bowl to a painting.

January 21. It is almost spring outside. The sun is shining and the day has an anticipation of early spring—a sense of secret stirrings in every tree and bush. Today as I was sitting by the window, the day stretching before me, I felt a burst of happiness and contentment. It is a pleasure to be here, in my own home and to have a baby on the way.

The baby is now moving and pushing its feet and hands out quite vehemently. How strange it is not to know what it looks like. Tom and I started the process, but we have no say in the result. Will it have my long fingers and toes? Will it have Tom's light brown hair and darker eyebrows? Will it have my short broad nose or Tom's distinguished aquiline nose—or neither? When the baby is older, will it be like Tom and me and love literature but run the other way when math is mentioned? Even though we cannot answer a single question about what our baby will be like, we know we will love it. It will not be a stranger. The bonding process between myself and the baby has already started. I am already becoming motherly.

Sometimes I wonder how a person from another planet where reproduction occurred differently would view pregnancy. The entire process would seem bizarre. I am a person with another person growing inside me. That other person does not begin large and diminish in size in order to fit through the small opening it has to pass through (like Winnie the Pooh getting stuck in Rabbit's door and having to stay there until he can lose enough weight to fit through). Instead, the baby grows larger and larger. When it is ready, my body will stretch to accommodate it.

My body is completely at the service of this baby. If I did not take in enough nutrients for the baby and myself, the baby would take them from my body. It is my body, not my mind, which has been at the baby's service all along. Sometimes I wonder if I have much to do with the process. Can I say I am growing this baby when my body is doing the nurturing without conscious effort on my part? Yet I cannot separate my mind and body.

The first nine months of a baby's life are essentially taken care of if the mother takes care of herself. It is as if God wanted to give the baby a good start, then transfers responsibility to the mother, though the child is always ultimately God's child.

I say I do not know this baby yet, but as I think about it, I realize that I do know it in a certain way. I know it now the way I know God. In prayer, I do not see God, but I know he is there and often experience his presence. So it is with the baby. I do not see it, but I experience a communion with it. This is the special privilege of a mother. The father has to wait until the baby is there before he can know it.

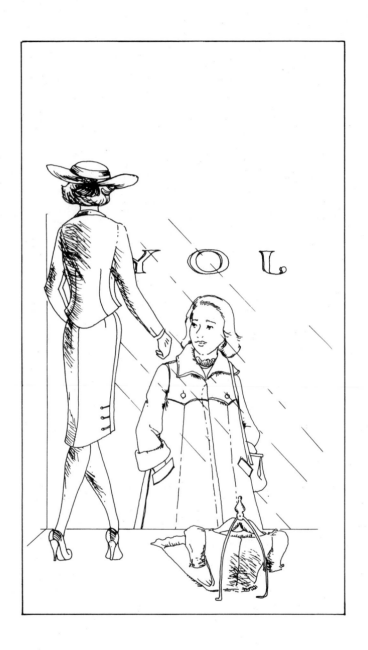

I feel about the baby the way I would feel about a present I was not to open. If the giver were special to me, I would carry the present with me and whenever I thought of it, I would feel a special happiness. This baby is a gift from Tom to me and me to him, and it is more than that, a new being, a person to be loved for itself.

I still am trying hard to stay away from sweets and carbohydrates, but it is difficult. I do not want to be fat after the delivery. I dream of wearing clothes with waists. Waist? What is that? At present I constantly bump into people and doors because I cannot correctly judge my size.

My most recent reading (aside from my escapist detective stories) is on breastfeeding. The things women have to go through to have a baby! The number of things that make us feel awkward and foolish! Consider the nursing bra. I think when I look at the size of what I have to buy, "How could I be that size?" I read about rubbing my nipples with a towel to toughen them—about the thick yellow lanolin I must rub on them that will not wash off; about the soreness when my milk comes in, so much that I will not be able to lie on my stomach; about the way my breasts may leak in public and leave two big wet spots on my dress; about the problems of breastfeeding in public; about using something that looks like a bicycle horn to pump my breasts; about the baby biting me when it grows teeth. Why, I ask, why put myself through all this? Yet this is part of life for women. It is (I cannot believe it) normal. Most women enjoy breastfeeding!

January 22.   How slowly the days drag by. I am working part time at the tailor's shop. I worked today and will work again on Thursday. The rack is filled with suits to be altered, so I can work as much as I want to. Working does help pass the time.

Today at work I listened to a radio discussion about

abortion. Four people were presenting their case for the freedom of women to choose abortion. My thoughts about abortion are changing. Until I became pregnant I had no strong feeling about it one way or another. I could understand women who felt they could not handle pregnancy, and I could also understand the position of those who thought abortion is wrong.

Now I have a harder time seeing justifiable reasons for abortion. I think each woman is responsible for the life that begins in her body, and I think the men who help to create this life are responsible, too. Once we initiate the process of life, something sacred has begun. Although it is not visible and our bodies rather than our conscious minds nurture it, it is there, sacred and demanding, a gift of God.

Expediency is the main reason for abortions, with the exception of abortions for medical reasons. Jesus was killed for purposes of expediency. Death was the easiest way to silence him.

As I write this, I am aware that I am speaking from a privileged position. I have a husband who loves me. We have enough money to support a child. We have room in our house. I know many people who contemplate abortion have none of these things. It appears to them to be the only solution. I can easily understand their desperation. Still, I cannot accept it. An action can make perfect sense but still be wrong.

Time to go to sleep now. I do not look forward to going to bed. At night I feel as though a clock is ticking in my head, and I am aware of each hour passing. The morning is always a relief.

January 23.   I am surprised to see how much the pile of yellow pages is growing as I write. The writing has helped clarify my thoughts. I know now that I am worried about how well I will adjust to having a baby and to the role of mother. The awareness is good. Understanding my concerns makes it easier to discuss them with Tom. The writing does more than help me to worry better, though. It gives me a small but significant sense of accomplishment each day.

Last night I had a spell of crying because I felt that Tom was tired of me; I was not attractive to him; I was too big and ugly-looking. It was an overreaction, perhaps from the fatigue of working all day. I am experiencing great insecurity about my appearance during this last month. I want to be back to my normal size. I wonder how long the return to normalcy will take.

I try to spend at least half an hour in the morning praying. I have been trying to be more appreciative of my life as it is right now and the way God is working in it. This morning I spent the first ten minutes thanking God for his blessings. As I did so, I felt increasingly happy. Many things came to mind to be thankful for. What struck me most was the fact that God has been faithful to me. Since the time ten years ago when I asked him to come into my life, he has not left me, even though I have often ignored him or drifted away from him. Thinking of his constancy was a comforting thought, a buoy in the shifting tides of the day.

God is faithful. Something of his nature has been revealed to me. Knowing God's nature gives me peace. I am reminded that as Christians we are in a covenant relationship with God. He will not break his covenant: "Deep within them I will plant my Law, writing it on their hearts. Then I will be their God and they shall be my people" (Jer. 31:33).

Love is something else to meditate on. It is at the heart of marriage and children. I can plan and prepare and talk and write and think, but love is what makes my life work. A strange thing, love. I don't think Tom's and my love for each other will be diminished by the addition of another person. Apparently, many women are afraid that children will diminish their relationships with their husbands. Love multiplies. It grows to fit the needs. Children should increase the atmosphere of love in our home—they should add to the presence of God, who is love.

January 25. I was not motivated to write today. I did everything else but write—vacuumed the house, defrosted the refrigerator, took a nap, made a shopping list, and walked downtown.

It is easy to get used to this life of not working, although there will be changes when the baby comes. I love the quiet when I am alone. Even the record player disturbs me. I would rather hear the sounds of the house creaking, the heat turning on and off, the mailman coming to the door, and the wind outside.

I am making small places of beauty in the house. I have brought a small piece of the season inside, a bare branch with a few red berries still clinging to it. Something new and lovely has been added to the room. My sister-in-law used to teach a class of difficult-to-handle children in New York City. She brought something new and beautiful into the room each day and asked the children to find it. The exercise made them appreciative of their environment and aware of the beauty that surrounds all of us.

How can I be a loving wife when I have to get up in the night to feed the baby? I was so grouchy this morning from not sleeping well that I could not stand to be around myself.

There is nothing I am not sensitive about lately, especially in regard to Tom. The smallest word or tone of voice makes me suspect he does not love me. On some days he seems like a stranger, and I seem like a stranger to myself.

Another Lamaze class yesterday. Two couples were absent. One, it turned out, had their baby. Unfortunately, the wife had to have a Cesarean section because she never dilated beyond one centimeter after her water broke. The instructor said that, on the average, one person in each class has a Cesarean. I hope this means the quota is filled in my class.

We practiced breathing techniques for pushing the baby out. For pushing, the mother lies on her back with her knees bent and cupped in her hands, legs as far apart as possible, or she lies on her side with one leg pulled up. The latter is more comfortable in practice. I found both positions embarrassing.

One of my favorite drawings in *The Little Prince* is of a snake who has swallowed an elephant. He looks like a side view of a cowboy hat: flat at the brim, then up in a big hump, then flat again. Now I know not only what the snake looked like, but what he felt like. Once the snake swallowed that elephant, he was no longer a graceful, quick, lithe creature anymore. In fact, he probably had trouble moving at all. That is me. If someone drew me, I would look like the snake turned on end.

One perverse pleasure of the Lamaze class is seeing others in the same position as myself. When we lie on the floor to do the breathing exercises, my own grunts and panting mingle with those of my classmates. There are seven of them. They all grumble about backaches, restless nights, heartburn, pants that slide down, and friends who begin their conversations with, "Boy, are you getting big!"

January 26. I am sitting in front of a fire. It has been a long time since we had one. The wood, which dried in our side yard through spring, summer, and fall, is burning fast. It sounds like tin foil being crushed and uncrushed.

I watch the flames consume the logs and consider how quickly my days pass by, consumed by petty pursuits. Tom and I ran errands all day, but I feel no sense of accomplishment. How terrible it would be to come to the end of life and feel that way. "Teach us to count how few days we have and so gain wisdom of heart," wrote the psalmist (90:12).

I am rereading Malcolm Muggeridge's *Something Beautiful for God*. It is his account of the work of Mother Theresa of Calcutta, a Catholic nun who left a comfortable life to work among the sick and dying in India. She instituted an order of nuns called the Missionaries of Charity. Her life challenges me to think about what I am doing with my life and to consider how generous I am being with it. It also provides food for thought on the issues of abortion and euthanasia. Mother Theresa is a contradiction of the values of modern society. Her actions say that life is not expendable, that those lives not useful to society are still valuable, that we have no right to do away with a life that is not convenient or does not serve our purposes.

Along with the Jews who were killed during World War II in Germany, great numbers of elderly and mentally or physically ill persons were also put to death. Because they did not fit in the Nazis' master plan, killing them was the quickest and easiest way of solving the problem.

In India overpopulation is a major problem. When someone dies neglected in the street, the tragedy is often dismissed—one less mouth to feed. Mother Theresa sees the starving and neglected poor as individuals and cares for them as such. She believes that whenever she touches a person, she is touching the body of Christ.

Reality. Living in reality is seeing the spiritual as well as the physical dimension of life. If the physical were all there is to life, then we could have value only to the degree that we were useful to one another. Our real value, though, is measured by our value in the sight of God.

January 28. This afternoon I see the doctor again. I have some questions for her: what do I take for heartburn? When do I go to the hospital? Will the doctor do an episiotomy even if it does not seem urgently needed?

Today life seems hard. I wish it were summer and I were twelve years old again, lying on a hill by myself. Why is it necessary to grow up and become serious about everything? Will there ever be another carefree day?

Nature is vast and profound, but it is busy about just one thing: being. It is always changing, but never changes. It has accepted its seasons of coming and going, of skeletal winter and spring brilliancy. It is reasonable and knows life is made up of seasons. Me—I want to be naked when I am clothed and clothed when I am naked. Part of me cries out for one thing at the same time that another part of me wants the opposite. In the morning I am elated, and in the evening I am depressed. Yesterday I celebrated friendship. Today I wish I were a hermit. I am reminded of a poem by Wendell Berry called "The Peace of Wild Things":

When despair for the world grows in me
and I wake in the night at the least sound
in fear of what my life and my children's lives may be,
I go and lie down where the wood drake
rests in his beauty on the water, and the great heron feeds.
I come into the peace of wild things
who do not tax their lives with forethought
of grief. I come into the presence of still water.
And I feel above me the day-blind stars
waiting with their light. For a time
I rest in the grace of the world, and am free.

47

A good poem should be good when you read it again in five years and in ten years. It should shimmer with new shades and intensities of meaning each time it is read. "The Peace of Wild Things" has worn well since I first found it several years ago.

The limits of my thoughts about God are widened to know that he created beings who could do something so mysterious and indefinable as writing poetry. He is larger than I can grasp—more whimsical, more full of beauty.

Writing is almost a form of weaving, picking up loose threads from the past, the present, and the future—blending them together. It is satisfying work. More enjoyable to me than weaving could be, but then I like observation and vicarious experience more than direct experience.

> I am the antennae of a moth,
>   A filter tasting the air,
>   A radio receiving signals,
>   A weather vane turning with the wind.
> I am a cat's whiskers. I am.

January 29.   The word *vulnerable* keeps running through my mind. I wish I could communicate more adequately to Tom. I need attention and tenderness, but this is one of his busiest times at work and his mind is elsewhere.

Walking down the street to buy some pineapple chunks to make sweet and sour pork for dinner, I thought for the hundredth time how strange it is to be pregnant. That has been a common thought from the beginning. I never thought it would happen to me, only to other women. Sometimes it is difficult to connect my inner reality with the outer, my mind and spirit with my body. I keep telling myself, yes, it is true.

By being pregnant, I am suddenly thrust on stage. Sometimes I have pretended it is happening to someone else—not a very healthy attitude. The outer woman puts on her costume, while the inner woman retreats to a safe place. When we are young, we have safe places like our parents' arms or our beds. When we are older, we still need safe places, but they are not always physical places. I have physical safe places, like the room I use for my study or my bed or next to Tom, but I also have an interior safe place. Sometimes I retreat to that interior place to get away from what is happening outside myself, but often it is to be with the Lord and to draw strength from him. Like the ocean, I need a balance of advance and retreat, of inner life and outer. Not that the boundaries are easily defined, for one flows into the other, but there are times for each.

Another trip to the doctor. It has been so long since I had seen my particular doctor that I could not remember what she looks like. I sat in the waiting room reading magazines and trying to remember her face. I read an article on Cesareans and the negative feelings women experience after a Cesarean; an article on a child born retarded and sent to a home for retarded children; an article on amniocentesis (testing the amniotic fluid) and the risks involved. All calculated to make this expectant mother sweat while waiting for the doctor's summons.

Once I saw her, I remembered her: short-cropped, slightly masculine hairstyle, large glasses, and a friendly, nonmedical manner. If asked to guess her occupation from a shapshot, I would pick something like physical education rather than medicine. A girls' hockey coach. I hope she delivers the baby, though I probably will not care which doctor is in charge when the time comes.

The examination showed that the baby's head is down, and it will probably drop farther into my pelvis in a week or so. I now must visit the office every week. I had only gained a quarter of a pound in the last two weeks. Happiness! Especially since I have been averaging four to five pounds a month. One month left to hold the line. I want to get back into my old clothes. The novelty of being pregnant is wearing off.

Prayer has been hard lately. It is difficult to keep my mind focused on one topic for more than two minutes. I leave church and cannot remember what the sermon was about.

January 31. I am rereading a book by the Italian journalist Oriani Fallaci called *Letter to a Child Never Born*. It is in the form of a letter from a mother to the child in her womb. I am not sure whether it is a true story or not. The dust jacket calls it a novel, but it reads like autobiography. The woman in the book is not married, is a successful journalist, and learns she is pregnant. She tries for weeks to decide whether to keep the child or not. One day she happens to see a picture of a three-week old fetus in a magazine, and her decision is made. She will keep it.

Though I come from a world very different from Oriani Fallaci's, I can see that many of the thoughts and feelings of expectant mothers are universal. Consider her reflections on the fact that men cannot bear children:

Is that an advantage or a disadvantage? Up until yesterday it seemed to me an advantage, even a privilege. Today it seems to me a limitation, even an impoverishment. There's something glorious about enclosing another life in your own body, in knowing yourself to be two instead of one. At moments you're even invaded by a sense of triumph, and in the serenity accompanying that triumph nothing bothers you: neither the physical pain you'll have to face, nor the work you'll have to sacrifice, nor the freedom you'll have to give up.

No woman would endure the discomfort and changes of pregnancy if they were not basically satisfying and fulfilling experiences.

Last night I went on a tour of the hospital. I had imagined labor rooms full of important-looking equipment. Actually they look very ordinary. Each has two beds, flowered curtains, a bathroom and shower. The large recovery room was also disappointing, containing several beds which each can be made private by curtains that enclose them. The nurse who gave me the tour was efficient and matter-of-fact. She had probably given the tour a hundred times. The whole experience made childbirth seem somehow mundane and mechanical. In the myriad of rooms, everyone has a job; every object has its function. The mother's function is to arrive on time and produce a baby.

I am reminded of a fascinating visit Tom and I made to a Hutterite community called the Bruderhof (German for "Brotherhood"). We stayed for a weekend. The community originated in Germany in 1920, but was forced to leave as Hitler gained power. The Bruderhof is self-sufficient, producing wooden toys called Community Playthings. There are three communities, each with about two hundred members.

When we arrived we found a welcome sign on the door of our room. On the bureau was a basket filled with candy, oranges, and soft drinks. Behind the basket were pictures drawn for us by community children. One had my name on it, and one had Tom's name on it. Of all the memories I carried away from our stay, the habit of greeting visitors with gifts and art work stands out most vividly. I wish some of the spirit of the Bruderhof could be found in hospitals, a personal touch that would say, "You are special; we know this is a special time for you." I understand why some women choose to have their babies at home.

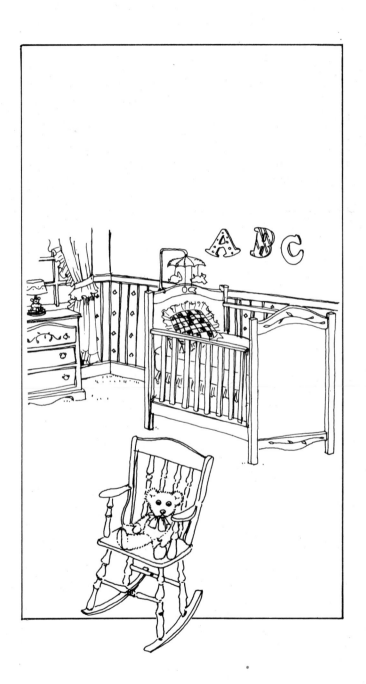

Yesterday I started sewing for the baby's room. It is a fine feeling to begin making the room look like a welcoming place. I made a quilted pad for the top of the changing table and some sheets for the cherry wood cradle my father made. I paid a price for crawling around on the floor cutting the material. Later in the day I had a number of Braxton-Hicks contractions (contractions which occur periodically during pregnancy, but do not increase in strength and regularity), more uncomfortable ones than I have had so far, and I tossed and turned all night trying to find a good position. I should have started sewing three months ago.

Tom has gone out of town for three days on business. I explained to him yesterday that I was feeling vulnerable and that I needed more of his attention. He understood. Perhaps I am becoming too self-centered, pampering myself too much. I don't know.

Today is the last day of January. Suddenly I am sad the month has gone. February marks the end of my term, and the weeks will probably pass quickly. There is no turning back.

February

February 1. Women writers are flourishing these days, but many are bent on pounding home this or that hard-line ideology. Each has her own soapbox, and the shouting sometimes drowns out the valuable things she has to say. We need women writers who can express the full complexity of women's lives—passionately, but also with clarity and without bitterness. It is easy to condemn, to concentrate on the mud at our feet; it takes vision to see the mountains toward which we are moving.

I grew up with the idea that being bored was my own fault. I still believe that and more—that being miserable is often our own fault. Life offers a multitude of possibilities, even within the limitations of any real situation, but it takes immense effort to deal constructively with a situation.

I am struck as I read *The Irrational Season* by Madeleine L'Engle, by the way her life and thoughts revolve around the Gospel. That is what my life should do. That is where the challenge and the joy of life should spring from—that so rich seed, which once planted, will never stop growing.

When Tom was an orderly, he worked with a priest named Father Michael. Father Michael was in his eighties, and so afflicted by Parkinson's disease that he could not control the continuous shaking of his body. Many of the men in the Care Center where Tom worked had become bitter or mean because of their suffering. Not Father Michael. He was considered by many to be a holy man. It was reported he had healed the sight of another priest by praying over him. Father Michael read and reread his large-print edition of the New Testament. This was his chief occupation. It was also his chief consolation, and he never became bitter or complained.

February 2. Little by little I am making the baby's room ready. Today I made a plastic cover for the cradle mattress, some fitted sheets, and some bumper pads. Next I will make wall hangings with pockets in them to hold things like diaper pins, shampoo, thermometer, etc. Doing these small things makes me feel that I am welcoming the baby into our life. "There is a room ready for you in this house, Baby, and there is room for you in our lives. Come in. The time is ripe. The world will not be a cold and sterile place. There will be warmth and comfort, a father and a mother prepared to love you."

I want the baby to come at the right time. It is a tendency of mine to want to hurry events, to be concerned about what the future will bring, to be impatient with the present. All ways of not following God. In following God, time takes on new dimensions. The present becomes important because it is in the present that God works in our lives. There is no rushing him. God's things happen in the fullness of time, when the right preparations have been made.

Each step along the way is as important as the end. Cooperating with God is living at peace in the present. That does not mean living passively. It means listening, for the sound of his footfall, for his action in the present moment. We need to be more adept at savoring moments, being aware of their unique flavor and quality.

I asked my friend, Rebecca, to coach me, but we have not had time to practice the breathing exercises. What would happen if I went into labor now?

Two years ago I coached Rebecca in the birth of her child. Tom and I have known Rebecca and her husband Peter for almost nine years. We all lived in Boston, were part of the same prayer group. Rebecca and Peter moved to Ann Arbor to be part of a more committed Christian group, and we moved here for the same reason six months later.

Rebecca and I have totally different personalities. She is

outgoing and bold; I am more reserved and cautious. Some of her best qualities seem at first to be faults. She can be so candid that she hurts people's feelings, but everyone knows exactly what she thinks. People immediately feel part of her life. She angers easily, but she is quick to forgive and readily sees what needs to change in herself. She has a largeness of spirit that says there is room in her life for other people. Our friendship has taken time to develop, but it has been solidified by the many experiences we have shared.

I had thought Rebecca was joking when she told me she was going to have her baby at home. It was not a joke. Peter would deliver the baby, with a doctor present in case of emergencies.

Since Peter would be busy with the delivery, I was asked to coach Rebecca. I wasn't sure I wanted to. I wasn't sure it was wise for Rebecca to have the baby at home, and I wasn't sure I could be a good coach since I had never gone through labor myself. There was another, more selfish reason: I didn't want to spoil the experience for myself. I was afraid pregnancy would seem commonplace after the Lamaze classes and the coaching. In the end I decided to coach her because I wanted to support Rebecca.

Peter and Rebecca first considered having the baby at home because they did not have health insurance. After looking into it more fully however, they decided they would have wanted to have the baby at home regardless. They consider the home environment better for mother and baby than that of an impersonal hospital. They had other children, and they also decided that home childbirth was a natural and healthy way to introduce the new baby into the family. The birth went well, and they never regretted the decision. When my own time came, Tom and I felt more comfortable with the conventional way of having babies in the hospital.

Rebecca and I started her Lamaze classes on a snowy February night two years ago. They were a revelation to me. I found I knew almost nothing about what happens physically to a woman during childbirth. It was fascinating. During the class I developed an intense desire to be pregnant myself, though I did not actually become pregnant until a year later.

We went faithfully to the six classes, enduring more snowy nights, then waited. I called Rebecca daily to see if anything was happening. Did she feel a spurt of energy? Did she think the baby had dropped? Had she lost her mucous plug? Nothing. I jumped for the phone whenever it rang. Two days before the due date at about seven in the morning, Rebecca's call finally came. Tom had never seemed so slow. He kept telling me there was no rush, but I was afraid I would miss the birth.

I had nothing to fear. The labor progressed rapidly at first (the doctor declared at nine that the baby would be born by noon), but then labor slowed down. By 6 o'clock Rebecca had only dilated to six centimeters. People came and went through the house in a great bustle. Meanwhile, I stayed with Rebecca and coached her. At almost the climax of Rebecca's labor a man from the CIA knocked on the door. He was gathering information about a young man who had lived with Peter and Rebecca and had applied for a job with the agency. After looking around, he asked, "Is someone here having a baby or something?" Peter was wearing a hospital gown. The doctor was sitting on the couch. I was walking up and down the room with Rebecca. It felt like a scene from a bad novel.

The baby came at an awkward angle and was caught on the lip of the cervix. As it pushed, it bruised the cervix and prevented full dilation. At about nine in the evening, the cervix finally dilated and a head appeared followed by the body of a baby girl. I started to cry—the baby had arrived, safe and healthy, a new person. She might have been my own, so relieved and exalted did I feel. Undaunted by suddenly finding herself out in the world, she gasped, blinked her eyes a few times, managed to get her thumb in her mouth, and was soon asleep.

True drama is supposed to be a cathartic or cleansing experience. I had been part of one of the most fundamental of human dramas—birth. Though I was tired and hungry, I also felt cleansed and renewed.

February 3. In *The Irrational Season*, Madeleine L'Engle discusses two Greek words that refer to time. One is *kairos*, which the biblical writers use to refer to God's time: a perpetual, self-forgetting present. The other is *chronos*: our time, chronological time. These terms sort out my thoughts about time in relation to God. Heaven will be *kairos*, an eternal present. Sometimes I experience a sense of *kairos* when I am praying. Then I feel prayer as joy and could go on and on with it. At other times I am bogged down in *chronos* and each minute I pray seems like an hour.

I tried to go to sleep tonight, but I couldn't because I had avoided writing. I had avoided my pad of yellow sheets, letting it intimidate me. I have to fight against my fears of inadequacy. I forget these fears for days—sometimes weeks, and suddenly they return, just to show me I haven't gotten rid of them. On Wednesday there will be a baby shower. I am nervous about being the center of attention, not sure I will say the right things, afraid people will come out of a sense of duty. The beast timidity again. Useless —not to be given in to.

February 4. No position was comfortable in bed last night, but if I am uncomfortable, how must the baby feel? It must feel cramped. Today as I was sewing, it kicked so hard that I imagined small feet pushing out of my stomach.

Some books say that the baby plays an active part in commencing labor. E. K. Hess has done experiments with ducks that show that when the time comes for young to be hatched there is an interchange of vocalizations between the mother and the eggs. The mother's vocalizations help synchronize hatching and facilitate imprinting (attachment of the ducklings to their mother).

I whimsically wonder if talking to the person inside this big stomach will persuade it to come sooner. I would not be surprised if it sensed my readiness or lack of readiness and responded. What signs and signals do I unconsciously pass on to it?

I expect to be late in delivering this baby because my cycle is a long one (more than twenty-eight days). According to the experts, the longer the cycle the later the delivery tends to be. We will see.

I have had increasing numbers of Braxton-Hicks contractions. Today I was back at the tailor's shop, helping out with a sudden rush of work. Standing at the ironing board pressing open seams, I felt one contraction after another. I am much more aware of these contractions than I was three weeks ago. They are more intense and more frequent. In the middle of a task I become aware of something happening to my abdomen. When I touch my stomach, it is hard, as if I were tensing my stomach. The contraction feels like a belt suddenly being tightened. The real thing will probably feel the same way, but be far more intense. My body is practicing. How odd to think that even though my body has never done this before, I can, with a fair amount of assurance, trust it to do just the right things when the time comes.

I think of animal migration, something scientists

are just beginning to understand. At the right moment (what makes it right is one of the puzzles) the animal begins its journey, often over thousands of miles. Though the animal may never have traveled the course before, it knows its destination and almost always arrives. Some animals navigate by smell. Salmon travel down fresh water rivers to the ocean and return to the same rivers to spawn. They recognize their respective rivers by scent. Homing pigeons navigate by orientation to the magnetic fields of the earth. Some birds navigate by the sun, some by the moon. The common factor among these animals is that they all have built-in navigation systems. When the right time comes, their bodies urge them on to their journeys and bring them reliably to the right places.

I am developing a great respect for the human body. It is not merely "the flesh," the lesser half, to be trained and disciplined. The body is remarkably complicated, harmonious as a poem in the way all the parts are related, sturdy yet delicate and minutely sensitive.

Much of what the body does, it does without command or intervention, but it can also cooperate with the reasoning mind. The voluntary and involuntary activities are interrelated. I do not think the body evolved and was then designated as a temple for the Holy Spirit. I think it was planned from the beginning as a temple for the Spirit.

If the body was so well designed, why does it grow old and get sick and die? Why do trees live longer than humans do and buildings stand longer? We were not intended for built-in obsolescence. The inconsistency is striking: the wonder of the design and its fatal flaws.

Death is not simply a physical event. It is a change of being involving the whole man. The Bible does not distinguish sharply between spiritual death and physical death. That makes sense because I am continuous with my body. The part of me that is called "I" could not exist without the subconscious forces that shape it and the involuntary actions that take place in my body. The conscious "I" is a sum of things beyond the body as well as within it. If my spirit is in a state of spiritual death, my body will be subject to death. But if my spirit is alive in Christ, physical death will be an entry into a new and more glorious life.

The New Testament does not define eternal life as the immortality of the soul. It speaks of the resurrection of the body. There it is again, the indissolvability of body and soul. Then we will be as we were created to be: fully alive, fully in union with God, and in fellowship with one another.

"You shall love Yahweh your God with all your heart, with all your soul, with all your strength," says Deuteronomy (6:4-5). We are to love God with our whole being, and place ourselves fully in His care. Sometimes at night I have trouble going to sleep because I do not want to surrender consciousness. I do not trust that God will care for me when I cannot care for myself. Death is the last surrender, the total surrender, before coming at last into God's presence.

February 5. The first complication of the pregnancy so far—swollen ankles. I push with my finger on my ankle, and when I take my finger away, a dent remains. The nurse tells me to drink fluids to help my body rid itself of the wastes that are causing the buildup. I would have cut down on fluids. I am not uncomfortable because of the swelling, but I am a little surprised by it.

This morning I visited the dentist. A foolhardy thing to do in the ninth month of pregnancy, I discovered. The hygienist put me in a chair and tipped it back. Then she turned a bright, hot light right on my eyes and began lacerating my gums with her sharp picks. After fifteen minutes, I was sweating and on the verge of losing my breakfast. "Let me sit up," I begged her. The baby was resting on my stomach and backbone. The hygienist finished quickly, but not quickly enough for me.

February 6. I see many women who have just had babies, but very few provide me with the model I would like. Perhaps I am looking for a supermother. When I listen to women, I hear about the boredom of being trapped indoors, the difficulty of being self-disciplined about eating, the dullness of housework, the continual demands of a baby. A little of this complaining goes a long way. Isn't there a way of being a victorious housewife? I know some hardships are part of the sacrifice of being a mother and housewife, but aren't there creative ways of dealing with them?

I have some ideas about the kind of person I want to be as a mother (I will find out later how realistic they are). I want to be a person who is continually learning and finds interest in her children and their development. I want to have interests of my own: exercise, reading, writing, hobbies. I want to be strong enough to avoid being immobilized or dominated by my children, and involved enough with the world not to make my family the sole subject of my conversation. It would be easy to lose myself in motherhood to an unhealthy degree. It is better to maintain perspective. Lastly, I want to be a loving mother, and I want love to characterize my home.

I want to find ways while I am at home of receiving outside stimulation. There is reading and talking to other women. I also might be able to take evening classes.

Here I am again, trying to solve every problem before the baby comes. Good luck. Hopefully, having children will open new doors. So often we see only the doors that will close.

February 8. Another visit to the doctor. I knew I had been retaining fluids because my ankles were swollen, but I found out I had gained four pounds worth of fluids. The doctor said the weight gain is not worrisome because the end is near, but it bothers me. I feel bloated, and when I look at my ankles they look as though they belong to an old lady. Two tree trunks. Then I put on my maternity stockings, which are too long. They gather in ripples at my ankles. It is hard to feel feminine.

Last night a friend visited with her two-year-old son. "What are you the most afraid of in having a baby?" she asked me.

"Of everything I've heard from other mothers: being alone, being bored, having only a child to talk to all day. You name it, I'm afraid of it," I replied.

"You sound perfectly normal," she said. "But don't worry; you are creative—you have nothing to fear. You will have to make some adjustments, but when you have done that you will be surprised at how full and how challenging your life will be."

Those words of encouragement were very helpful.

The baby shower was splendid. After the first ten minutes I stopped pretending it was for someone else. I was touched by the number of handmade gifts I received. Everything from blankets to mobiles to stuffed animals. It was fun to bring the presents home and lay them out and admire each one. I spent a long time doing that, making piles and rearranging the piles. I didn't want to put them away. I wanted to leave them spread out over the couch and living room floor so that I could keep looking at them.

We had an inch of snow last night. It was the first snow of the winter, and it made me feel that winter had just arrived, although it is really almost over. I hadn't missed the snow. I was relieved that we didn't have to shovel the walk and dig out the car. But seeing the snow today reminds me of its special beauty. It is private, enclosing, softening, meditative, timeless. Each snowstorm has its own character, which depends upon the time of day it comes. Each storm makes time its captive, falling at a pace all its own, slowing the world's business.

February 10. Today the snow is gone. It never amounted to much by Michigan standards—a few flakes riding on the wind, slipperiness on the steps. If this were North Carolina where I grew up, I would not be surprised. Winter was short there. An inch of snow was enough to stop traffic and let the schools out.

After winter in North Carolina came a long and glorious spring. First came the sprays of Scotch broom, bright yellow on dark green, almost brown stalks. The ground would begin warming up, softening, and unleashing a tumult of smells: the smell of earth and moisture, the smell of flowers beginning to stir; crocuses, tulips, jonquils, daffodils, and pansies; and then there were the flowering trees: crab apple, pink and white dogwood—and redbud. The lawns were green by April and the birds had long since returned to claim last season's nests.

Spring was distinct from summer, when the heat bore down upon everything and the flowers hid to escape. People and animals slowed down and sought shelter in the shade. But spring was promise and renewal and jubilation. How can anyone understand the full meaning of rebirth without having experienced a North Carolina spring?

Here in Michigan spring sneaks in—a little sun one day, a few buds opening on a tree, a squishiness beneath the feet. Then one day, just as you are noticing the weather has become warmer, it is suddenly summer. The flowers are giving up after one or two bloomings. The ground thirsts for water and puts on its old brown coat almost before it has become green.

Logically people living in cold climates ought to view life as harsher (with less in it to celebrate) than people in warm climates. They should have a harder time believing in a kindly God and the benevolence of fellow human beings. Oddly enough, they don't. I have met just as many disgruntled southerners as serenely happy northerners.

I have a short memory for seasons. Whenever a new one comes, I am caught unawares, as if I had never experienced it before. I think, "I could not have stood another month of winter," though I am not aware of being unhappy with it until it is almost over. Spring is an appropriate time for a baby. I have never been a hiker but this spring I will begin. I will search out the small signs of change as spring progresses. I will start with barely noticeable phenomena: green buds, a green shoot sticking out of the earth, and I will trace these small changes until they become a crescendo of trees in bloom and flowers everywhere and grass up to the ankle.

The first spring I really noticed was when I taught nursery school. I wanted to teach the children to see what was around them, and I ended up learning myself. We went for a walk almost every day. One day we saw moss that had been covered by snow. Later we saw robins pecking in the softened earth for worms. Later still we moved some leaves and discovered the tender shoots of new grass growing. I don't know how much the children learned, but ever since then I have been an observer. Each season is busy preparing for the next. We experience abrupt changes, but the seasons are a steady progression. We are used to calendar thinking, with seasons beginning on a preordained day. That is *chronos*. The seasons go by *kairos*.

Perhaps I think so much about seasons because of the

season occurring within me. There is a process unfolding in me that has occurred millions of times before to others, but is miraculous to me in its precision and reliability. There is a progression of life to maturation, to ripeness, to reproduction, to full maturity, to death, to rebirth. Here I am, caught in the middle of it all, part of everything that is happening around me. When my baby comes, the trees around this house will be sprinkled with buds almost ready to unfold, announcing to all the world that there is new life, new hope—rebirth after a season of death.

February 12. The "Today" show reported on "Love American Style" in honor of Saint Valentine's Day. Reporters interviewed an unmarried couple who were living together. Their life-style was necessary because of the premises on which they based their lives. The woman said she distrusted marriage. She did not want to be boxed in or have to fit into a male-determined role. The man said their arrangement was practical. He was afraid of waking up in fifteen years and looking at his wife and thinking, "I don't know you." Both partners want to be certain they are right for each other before they get married, so they avoid commitment.

In a society where one out of two marriages ends in divorce, they are trying to be sure before taking the step. But living together before marriage is no assurance. One is bound to change over the course of years; one's partner will experience changes; one's circumstances in life will change. What is important to me is seeing marriage as a covenant made with one another before God. Our love is often flawed, but Tom and I know we can depend on God's grace where we are weak.

Why do I love Tom? This is like asking an actress to describe the scene in which she is acting. To do so she must stop acting and step outside the scene. She must take on an observer's role regarding a matter essentially subjective. Thomas Merton writes in *Disputed Questions*, "Love brings us into a relationship with an objectively existing reality, but because it is love it is able to bridge the gap between subject and object and commune in the subjectivity of the one loved." In other words I experience Tom as I experience myself, from my inwardness.

We are each made in the image and likeness of God, but we each reflect him in a unique way. I love many things about Tom, but they all hearken back to the essence of who he is. Tom reflects and concretizes God for me by being who he is. Something at the root of my being is attuned to and responds minutely to what is at the root of his being.

February 15.
It was you who created my inmost self.
and put me together in my mother's womb;
for all these mysteries I thank you:
for the wonder of myself, for the wonder of your works.

You know me through and through,
from having watched my bones take shape
when I was being formed in secret,
knitted together in the limbo of the womb.

(Ps. 139:13-16)

God is an artist, fascinated by the work of his hands. The psalmist acknowledges, "Yes, it was you, God, who created me, not just my body, but the totality of who I am. I am not a random combination of genes. I am a special entity. I am not the mechanical product of various processes. I am a creation."

Creation implies a creator, someone who took particular

care to have his creation turn out a certain way. The psalmist says, "You put me together": anatomy, personality, nature, everything. Then the psalmist thanks God. He is thanking God for creating him, but also for the fact that creation is a living mystery, not a cold mechanical process. What would life be without the mystery behind it? Each person can wonder at the miracle of his existence, the fact that out of all the possible gene combinations, his was the one that occurred.

No one, not even our parents, watched when we were being formed in the quiet darkness of the womb, like a tiny shoot breaking through its seed shell deep inside the ground. No one, the psalmist says, but God. The creator privately delights at what no one else can yet see.

In the darkness only God and the child exist. The womb: a place of safety where life is nurtured. A place in the world, but away from the world, where until recently no one could disturb the process taking place. God watches the bones take shape, writes the psalmist. What is happening is God's secret for a time. Only he knows what color the child's hair and eyes will be, whether the ears will stick out, or how big the nose will be.

We do not remember that time in the womb when all was darkness, but the faces of babies whose pictures have been taken in utero appear strangely peaceful. Perhaps it is a time of spiritual preparation for the shock to come. Perhaps when we are reunited with God after death we will know what that time before time was like. I do not see heaven as a return to the womb, safe and soft. At death we will be a composite of how we have spent our lives, but at birth we are new.

"Knitted together in the limbo of the womb." The heart, the lungs, the brain, the soul—are being knit together to work in harmony at birth. An exquisitely complicated process is taking place, much of which is not understood yet by scientists. Man is able to cooperate with and participate in creation, but he is not the creator.

Limbo implies a period in which time is motionless. There is no time for the fetus. No sun rising and setting, no hurrying, no befores and afters. All is a constant now. The baby experiences *kairos*, God's time. Life inside the womb is so qualitatively different from the rest of life that perhaps it should have a special name. We talk about afterlife; life in the womb might be called *forelife*, not meaning less than life, but rather life of a different quality.

Obviously there is no place where God is not, whether in forelife, life, or afterlife, unless we choose to exclude him. We are never created and then abandoned.

Since my due date is March 4, I could have the baby any time from the nineteenth of February to the eighteenth of March. Lent starts February 20. How appropriate to enter labor during the time commemorating Christ's suffering, death, and resurrection.

February 16.   It is late, about 1:00 A.M., but I can't go to sleep. It is as if there is some thought weighing on the edge of my mind that has to be articulated, something to do with the day just past.

As soon as Tom and I got home from dinner at a friend's house, I began to feel anxious. It started because my legs and ankles are swollen, then it became a wish that I wasn't pregnant, then a wish that I did not have to go through what lies ahead. Why did I get pregnant in the first place? I think of Christ in the garden of Gethsemane. He prayed that if possible, he be spared what lay ahead. He suffered but he continued to accept the will of the Father: "Let your will be done, not mine" (Luke 22:43). As I sit here uncomfortable, that thought comforts me. I hope the end is soon.

Heartburn, diarrhea, swelling. . . . I am ready for my old body again. I do not want to be brave or optimistic or anything else anymore. I want to be the old me. It's time for the baby to find a place of its own. It has been taking up more and more of my thoughts and my body. I need a little room.

I'll try to sleep now.

February 17. "How do you stand up to pain?" my friend asked me. I did not know how to answer. I have never experienced much physical suffering. Labor is a minor discomfort compared to the illness that some people manage to endure. I know a woman who has chronic arthritis. She is in constant pain, and yet she takes care of four young children. When I had the flu a week ago, I knew it would soon be over. Also, labor will have a foreseeable end. The woman with arthritis does not have that comfort. In fact, she knows that her illness will probably grow worse.

I do not want to write about suffering today. The sun is bright outside, and I am happy. I want to let some spring seep into this winterized mind. Each day warm weather gets closer. I see spring clothes in the stores. Beach and sand and sun seem like fantasies out of a children's fairy tale.

All of a sudden it is terribly hard to wait. Probably because I know that tomorrow is two weeks from the due date.

This morning was practice time for breathing techniques. I spent about an hour and a half practicing with Rebecca coaching me. In the Lamaze method, each stage of labor has a pattern of breathing that goes with it. I feel confident now of the techniques, but using them in the real situation will be different from practicing.

It is difficult to keep my distance from this event. When Tom comes home from work, I have to fight to take my mind off the baby and focus on him. Will it be more of a struggle

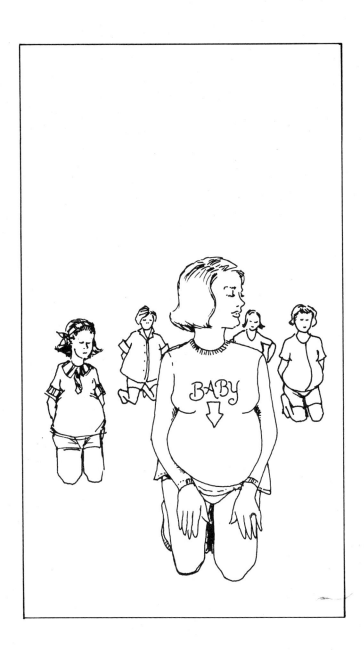

when the baby is actually here or will it become easier? Along with being parents, we will want to maintain an identity as a couple and as individuals, though an imbalance at first is probably unavoidable.

It is easy to become discouraged with writing. That must be the bane of most writers. We read a book and think, "I could never write anything like that." Of course not. Each person's style is different. I am easily intimidated by the vast plains of empty space in my mind when I sit down to write. It is amazing how quickly those spaces fill, though, when the words begin to come. The days I feel least inspired are sometimes the best for writing. How much more there is in our minds than we give ourselves credit for.

We continually fill our minds with outside stimuli—TV, books, magazines. For the last three nights I watched the Olympics on television. A seemingly innocuous pastime, but I noticed I was becoming increasingly passive, anesthetized. It does not matter what I am watching. The process itself is anesthetizing. I can drift off into a world without responsibility and without risk.

I think we all need to place ourselves in situations where we are afraid of failure. Those situations help us discover the resources we do have and the bounty God can supply. Like writing or any other creative art, prayer is risky: emptiness, waiting, experiencing our humanness, letting God fill us in his time. It is a creative emptiness—uncomfortable, easy to run from, subjecting ourselves to God's purpose, being changed (without realizing it) more into God's image, letting our hearts be enlarged, as Mother Theresa said, for God to fit in. I often do not want to pray. I find it hard to get beyond myself enough to see God. It is work, but I need the discipline. I need to know God's love as deeply as he wants to reveal it.

I should not be surprised that writing is part of the way to

God for me, yet I am. Why doesn't everyone else experience this call? It is another question like why God chose to make me rather than someone else; where did I come from in his mind? As surely as he chose me out of all the possibilities, I am going to be different and my way in life and my way to him will be unique.

God will not force me to follow him. I have to do it because I know it is right. Does what I am doing have any ultimate value? Does the bowl question the potter? I have to be the bowl I am made to be. There is a beauty in a tree standing in a field—being. There is a beauty in my doing what is right for me, a grace, a rightness that affects the rest of my life, a powerful peace. Doing the work I am called to do is a way of saying yes to God and living in his kingdom. That work may be ministering to the dying in the streets of Calcutta, as Mother Theresa does, or it may be raising children, or it may be working in a law office. The product is not always tangible; there is not always recognition.

Gerard Manley Hopkins wrote poetry for years, refusing to have it published during his lifetime. The brother who started the Little Brothers of Jesus labored many years among nomadic desert tribes. He had only one convert during his life, but later hundreds came to know God because of his work. Sometimes we don't see God's purposes but we still hear his voice and are invited to follow.

February 20. Ash Wednesday today, and a fitting day for it. The sky is bleak—it is damp—and yet there is the promise of spring in the melting snow. We went to mass and were marked by ashes with the sign of the cross on our foreheads. "From dust you came and to dust you shall return," the priest intoned as he crossed one forehead after another.

There was a comforting quality to those words, as if the

priest were saying, "You are what you are, nothing more, nothing less. The reality of life is that we will all die one day." The words put us all on the same level: the woman in her fur-collared coat and fashionable leather boots, the woman being pushed in the wheelchair, the family trying to pack nine bodies into one pew.

The guest editorialist in *Newsweek* this week wrote about Lent, pointing out that the more we have everything we need, the less we appreciate what we have. She said it was necessary for Americans, so used to instant gratification, to learn to deny themselves and thereby rediscover meanings that have been lost from their lives.

When Tom and I were newly married, we owned almost nothing. We were both in school and worked part time. We had only enough money for necessities. I remember feeling guilty for spending twenty-five cents on candy and debating long minutes at the grocery store over whether or not to buy a jar of pickles. Once I bought a lamp for twelve dollars and had to take it back the next day because we could not afford it. Poverty can be made to sound romantic. It wasn't, but it did help us to understand that the quality of our lives did not depend on material possessions. Since I stopped working we have been feeling the money pinch again, but I expect it to have beneficial effects.

February 21.   The news today is that there is no news. The doctor felt my cervix and said it was beginning to dilate. It has not flattened out yet. Also, she said the baby has not dropped into position for delivery with its head engaged in the pelvis. Distressing news, though I suspected as much. I have not felt any change, except that it gets continually harder to sleep and move around. February has been a long month. I will be glad when March finally arrives. The doctor said the baby would probably be late, maybe a week past the due date, which would put it around March 11th. I called my mother and told her not to pack her bags yet.

I don't want to put on any more weight in the next few weeks. I have already gained thirty pounds, five of which the doctor says is fluids. I try to eat moderately, but the pounds keep coming.

I am suddenly bored. Everything I can do to get ready is done. To keep myself busy, I will have to think up some new projects, but all my ambition has seeped away. At this moment nothing sounds better than bed and a good book. Withdrawal. I am depressed at what the doctor said.

It has taken us months to settle on names. We thought we liked a lot of names, but when it came down to giving a name to a baby for the rest of his life, none of them would do. Ruth or Joseph are the final choices. Unfortunately there is no way to consult the one most directly concerned. We will have to hope that he or she likes our choice.

Birth

Joseph Thomas O'Connor is now one day old! He weighed seven pounds, twelve ounces and was twenty-one inches long.

What happened is still hard for me to believe. . . . I had invited my sister for dinner. After dragging myself out of bed from an afternoon nap to fix dinner, I made a spinach quiche. After dinner we gathered in the living room to wait for my sister's roommate to arrive. The roommate came at 6:30. Barely had she sat down when I felt a small gush of water. I gave Tom a startled look, but I did not want to say that my water had broken. (The sac that surrounds the baby is filled with amniotic fluid; it often breaks and releases the fluid at the onset of labor.) I thought the baby might have been bouncing on my bladder. Tom said, "What's the matter?" Jokingly, my sister said, "Her water broke." I said, "I think it might have."

I went to the bathroom. When I sat down a stream of fluid came out, but I still was not sure. The fluid stopped. Then it started pouring down my legs, soaking my clothes. I was sure. I kept thinking, "This means I will have my baby by tomorrow."

My legs started shaking. I told everyone in the living room, and confusion broke loose. I tried to remember whether I had packed everything I needed in my suitcase and searched frantically for the piece of paper on which I had written the doctor's instructions in case my water broke. My sister and her friend tried to be helpful but only compounded the confusion. Everyone was bumping into everyone else. Eventually my sister and her friend left. I located my suitcase, and we called Rebecca (the coach) and the doctor. The doctor said to come to the hospital when the contractions were ten minutes apart.

Tom started timing the contractions. Some were five

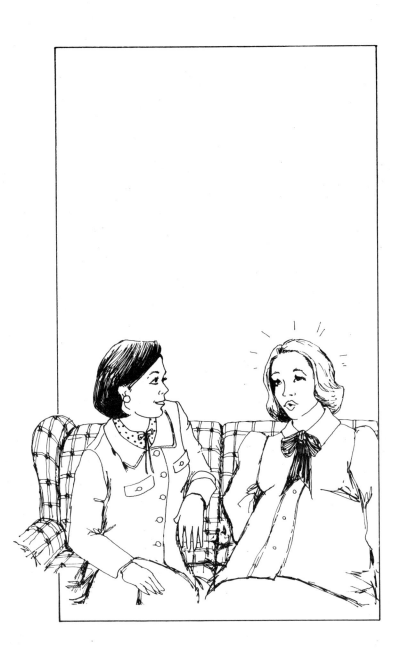

minutes apart, some were ten or fifteen minutes apart. I had a hard one, then several smaller ones. We decided to go to the hospital. The drive seemed longer than it ever had before. Rebecca and her husband Peter met us there.

That morning the doctor had said the cervix was beginning to open up and thin out. I realized that my body was not as ready as some women's are when they go into labor, because my cervix was only slightly dilated and effaced. It looked like a long labor. I could even imagine the necessity of a Cesarean section if the labor went too long.

When we arrived at the hospital we were sent to a labor room. A nurse came who was stamped out of the old battle-ax mold. She was a spare, graying woman dressed in scrub-room green, shoes covered with clear elastic plastic bags, hair in another plastic bag. Her appearance announced, "I've seen it all; you can't put anything over on me."

She checked to see how much I was dilated. It was about 8:30 P.M. then. I was dilated less than a centimeter out of the necessary ten (the width of four fingers together), but I had become almost totally effaced. My legs were still shaking. She folded her arms and looked me over. "It's going to be a long night," she said. "The fact that your legs are shaking means that you are nervous, probably because it's your first baby. You'll have to try to relax and take your mind off what you're feeling. Walk around. Forget about breathing techniques and timing contractions, because if you start that now the labor will seem a lot longer."

When I told her the contractions were painful, I needed the breathing exercises, and I did not feel like walking around, she said: "If you think the contractions are bad now, honey, just wait; they're going to get a lot worse. You aren't even in real labor yet because the contractions aren't coming at regular intervals and lasting sixty seconds."

78

When the resident came, he said they might send me home to get some rest before inducing labor in the morning. He said he would discuss it with my doctor.

Meanwhile I got into a hospital gown and robe, and we went out to the waiting room to rejoin Peter and Rebecca. I said to Rebecca, "If this isn't real labor, what is real labor like? I don't think I can take it." She reassured me, "This is the real thing. Those are good contractions you are having. It's just not going according to the book." That helped. Then we prayed together that the labor would progress quickly. Rebecca came into the labor room with me. At that point the resident suggested that I take a hot shower in the hope that it would speed up the labor.

I was in the shower for an hour. Despite the nurse's advice, I continued to do the breathing exercises. Deep breaths and relax. Breathe in through the nose on one, out through the mouth two, three. At the end of the contraction, take another deep breath, let it out and relax. For a focal point I chose the shower head. The contractions started coming with only a minute or two in between. I had not expected labor to be so intense and painful. When Rebecca had been in labor she was able to joke and talk. It was all I could do to stay on my feet, much less be civil. The shower, besides feeling wonderful, kept me out of view of the nurses and doctors.

At 10:30 the resident asked me to come out so he could check my progress. I had only dilated to one and one-half or two centimeters. He left the room and began discussing with Tom the possibility of a sedative to make me sleep through the night. The doctor thought I was overreacting to the contractions, but neither Tom nor the resident realized how hard and fast they were coming. While he talked, I crept back to the shower, where at least the shaking stopped. Tom told the doctor he did not think I needed a sedative. A good thing. Anyone who had tried to give me a sedative then would have heard in very unambiguous terms where to go with it.

Rebecca sat faithfully outside while I was in the shower. She timed the contractions and shouted encouragement. I came out briefly while the nurse tried to get a urine sample, and I was a glorious five centimeters dilated. Back in the shower, I could barely handle the contractions by myself. They were so hard, peaked so soon, and came so close together, that I began to suspect I was in transition (the most difficult part of labor, the last three centimeters of dilation).

Rebecca said she thought I should come out. I did. The nurse checked me, and I was eight centimeters dilated. The next contraction brought with it an overwhelming physical urge to push. The urge was uncontrollable, but I tried not to push because if the cervix is not fully dilated, it can be bruised by the pressure of the baby's head. The nurse assured me that it was all right to go ahead. With the first push the top of the baby's head appeared. No one was prepared for that. The resident ran in; Tom threw on a scrub gown; and together they wheeled the bed down the hall to the delivery room.

The delivery room was a white-tiled igloo ablaze with lights and filled with equipment. I had to slide off the bed onto a table where everyone started doing things to me at once. The anesthetist stuck an i.v. into my arm; the doctor simultaneously put my legs in the stirrups and put sterile coverings over them. The nurse was preparing me for the episiotomy. I felt like saying, "Why are you wasting time with all that? The baby's coming!"

With each contraction Rebecca helped me lean forward, and I pushed as hard as I could. After about three contractions the baby's head was out. I felt a stinging burning sensation, but other than that I could not tell what was happening. I did not feel the episiotomy when the doctor made the cut. All of a sudden it was over. The doctor lifted the baby, and it was a boy. I could not tell what his face looked like because his hair was plastered over his head. He was bluish, and he was covered with blood and the white vernix that keeps the baby's skin from becoming water-logged in the womb.

It was 1:00 A.M. Calm after the storm. The contractions stopped as soon as he was born. A few minutes later the placenta was delivered. I expected an onrush of maternal feelings toward my new baby or a feeling of joy or exhilaration. I felt nothing except relief that it was over.

From examining the placenta the doctor was able to tell that it had a terminal abruption—that is, part of the placenta had started pulling away from the wall of the uterus before the baby was delivered. The nurse had to suction some blood that the baby had swallowed in the womb. The doctor informed me that an abruption is not serious in itself, and not too uncommon, but a long labor could have been dangerous for the baby if the placenta had pulled away any more from the uterine wall and the baby had not been able to get enough oxygen. An abruption usually causes the labor to speed up. I wrote in an earlier section of this journal that I believed God would be with me in labor. I saw that he had been.

Tom watched as the nurse suctioned Joseph and cleaned him off. Later he told me that his first feeling had been pity toward the tiny helpless being that was his son. As soon as the nurse handed him to Tom, wrapped in a blanket, Tom asked that the lights be dimmed. Without the glare Joseph was able to open his eyes. Black, alert, seemingly perceptive, they stared up at Tom. A person revealed himself.

February 26.   My doctor arrived from a basketball game

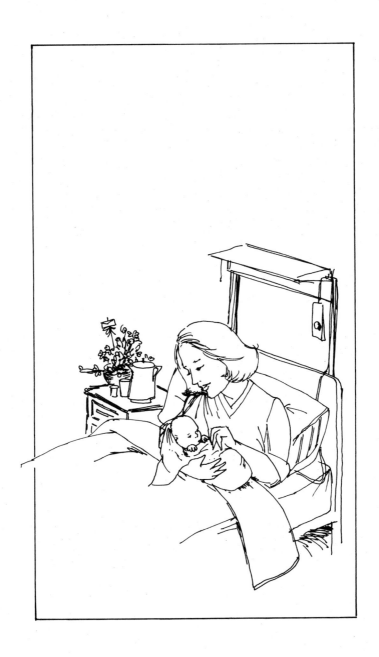

in time to sew up the episiotomy the resident had given me. That took about twenty minutes. From the delivery room I was wheeled to the recovery room, where I stayed two hours while my i.v. finished draining and the nurse kept checking my uterus to make sure it was contracting as it should. I was able to wheedle her into bringing me a Coke to quench my thirst. Then another nurse brought Joseph in, and I nursed him for the first time.

Some babies are not interested in nursing immediately after they are born. Not Joseph. He caught on right away. I still did not feel much toward him. Peter and Rebecca came in to see him, then they went home. Tom stayed with me until 3:00 A.M. when I was wheeled to my room. Joseph went back to the nursery.

The bed felt wonderfully warm and soft. It was a luxury to be able to lie on my back again after all those months. My first thoughts were of how glad I was not to be pregnant any more. I was grateful that it was all over. Then the wonder of what had happened began to roll over me.

When the nurse helped me into bed, she asked me if I wanted Joseph brought in for the 5 A.M. feeding. I told her I thought I wanted to sleep, but as I lay there, arms thrown back, expecting at any moment to fall asleep, my mind flooded with thoughts of Joseph and the miracle of birth.

The emotions I felt are difficult to label because they were such a mixture, but they were all positive. I was grateful for how well labor had gone, for the fact that I could be a mother, and for the particular baby we had received. I remembered what Joseph looked like with his dark and fuzzy head of hair, and how he had looked at me when I held him in the recovery room. I remembered the feel of holding him, and I wanted to hold him again. Suddenly 5:00 seemed interminably far away.

I felt the pride and good kind of tiredness that an athlete

feels after putting all his efforts toward a goal and winning. I was taking part in something larger than myself. Altogether it was a quiet sort of joy that I experienced lying there waiting for 5:00 to come. I never did sleep.

February 28. The stay in the hospital was pleasant and restful, and it gave me a few days respite before facing the task of caring for Joseph by myself. I stayed three days and came home on Monday morning.

I had not slept all night after Joseph was born, but I felt exhilarated in the morning. I showered and washed my hair, took sitz baths to ease the discomfort of the episiotomy, ate everything in sight, and rested in bed. Tom came to visit. We spent most of our time holding Joseph and staring at him.

Tom responded to Joseph more than I had expected he would. He wanted to hold him, wanted me to take pictures of the two of them and worried over whether Joseph was hot or cold. I couldn't relax while Tom was there. He called our families and enjoyed jolting them with, "It's a boy!" My mother must have been surprised because I had called her Thursday afternoon to tell her that I probably would not have the baby until around March 11. Three hours after we talked, my water broke.

Typically, Tom had thought all along the baby would be a boy, and I had thought it would be a girl. He kept looking at Joseph during his visit to see if there was any resemblance to him. It is hard to tell, but I think Joseph has Tom's hands and hair (including sideburns and widow's peak), and my feet and olive skin coloring.

On Sunday night while I was still in the hospital, Tom called my sister around 11 P.M. and said, "I don't have anyone to talk to about my son. Can you come over?" So my sister, obviously of a generous nature, drove over and stayed up with him until past midnight listening to him rave about his new son.

I was never extremely uncomfortable after the birth. The episiotomy was relatively small and healed nicely. Since I did not have any anesthesia, I did not have any uncomfortable side-effects from that. Nurses came around offering pain medication several times each day, but after the first night I did not need any.

I met the woman in the room next to mine. She also had dilated in a speedy six hours, but then she had to push for two. Finally the doctor literally had to pull the baby out with forceps. Even with an episiotomy she tore the muscle wall of her rectum. Her hospital stay was going to be a week or more. I was lucky. Three or four pushes and Joseph was out.

I am remembering the passage in which Jesus compares the apostles' feelings about his death to the way a woman experiences labor:

"I tell you most solemnly,
you will be weeping and wailing
while the world will rejoice;
you will be sorrowful,
but your sorrow will turn to joy.
A woman in childbirth suffers,
because her time has come;
but when she has given birth to the child she forgets the suffering
in her joy that a man has been born into the world.
So it is with you: you are sad now,
but I shall see you again, and your hearts will be full of joy,
and that joy no one shall take from you."

(John 16:20-22)

I cannot remember what the pain of labor felt like, although I know it was painful. That memory is replaced with joy at the presence of Joseph in our life and the wonder of who he is. Now I have some sense of what it will be like to leave this life and see Jesus face-to-face. The sorrows of this life will be forgotten in the joy we experience.

Another passage that had meaning for me in the hospital was Psalm 91:11-12—"He will put you in his angels' charge to guard you wherever you go. They will support you on their hands in case you hurt your foot against a stone." That was my labor. I felt protected from all the things that could have made it longer and more difficult.

The night before I came home from the hospital my faith faltered. I worried about every detail from how to dress Joseph to whether I would be able to care for him correctly. In order to rest before going home, I did not keep Joseph in my room at the hospital. He stayed in the nursery and was brought to me every four hours to be nursed. Of course I could go to him any time I wanted or keep him after a feeding for as long as I wanted. The only time he could not be in the room was during visiting hours.

To pick Joseph up I had to wash my hands with alcohol wipes. If Tom wanted to hold him, he had to put on a surgical gown. What are all the precautions for? What are they protecting the baby from, when in a day or two the baby will be home, and there will be none of these precautions?

I slept badly the night before leaving the hospital. In the early morning hours I lay awake wishing I did not have to go home and face the care of this child myself. The nurses were so competent. I did not even know how to give an infant a bath. What if he cried and I did not know how to make him stop? I had tried keeping him in the room one night. He made noises and woke up crying every hour or so. Finally at midnight, I shuffled down to the nursery with him and shamefacedly handed him back to the nurses.

My mother flew in from Washington on Monday morning and was met by my sister. Then they came to collect Joseph and me at the hospital. That morning I put on regular clothes for the first time since the birth. The swelling in my legs and ankles was gone. I was not back to my before-pregnancy size, but I was so much smaller than I had been of late that I actually felt thin.

The elaborate precautions continued until the last minute. I was not allowed to clothe Joseph myself to take him home. I laid out the clothes, then the nurse dressed him. I was not allowed to carry him downstairs myself. The nurse carried him and then handed him to me once I was inside the car. I watched her trim white figure disappear into the hospital and the automatic sliding doors close noiselessly behind her. Germs floated tangibly in the air around me. There was no protection now. Joseph was a tiny person in a huge world of potential dangers.

March

March 2.   The days are passing quickly. I grab at them, trying to get them down on paper. On the surface they appear uneventful, a succession of feedings, diaperings, and baths. I had no idea such simple activities could be so intense.

The first thing I noticed when we got back from the hospital was the dust on the windowsills in Joseph's room. It had to be removed immediately. My mother seemed to understand. She got a cloth and wiped the sills spotless while I removed the six layers of clothes I had brought Joseph home in. When I saw how the pajamas he wore hung on him I felt like crying. I had nothing small enough to fit him. My mother slipped a brightly wrapped present out of her suitcase. It contained two tiny stretch-pajama suits. They fit him perfectly.

My sister made some chicken sandwiches. I sat down gingerly in the rocking chair. Joseph was asleep. Maybe home wasn't so bad after all.

It was all trial and error that first day and night, mostly error. At night I put a gown on Joseph that tied at the bottom and put him in a cradle with a receiving blanket tucked over him, just as I had seen done at the hospital. I did not put rubber pants on over his disposable diapers. That night confirmed all my worst fears. He woke up every hour or two. I changed him completely three times and the last time he wet through the sheet too. Finally, I was so tired when he woke up again about 5:30 A.M. that I let him cry for a while. Mom, sleeping in the next room, got up, wrapped him in blankets and had him quiet in no time.

The doctor told me not to feed him more than every two and a half hours, so I tried not to nurse him too often. I couldn't understand why he was crying. Eventually I learned that I could put rubber pants on over his disposable diapers to keep his clothes dry, that he needed more blankets in our drafty apartment, and that he needed his feet kept warm with socks or booties if he did not have a pajama suit on. I also learned that the first night home from the hospital can be difficult for a baby because of the new environment. Fortunately Joseph decided on a four-hour schedule that first day and has stayed on it ever since.

I was grateful for my mother's presence. She enjoyed Joseph greatly, which helped me to enjoy him. One day she bought insulated curtains to make his room warmer plus treats for us, like cheeses and crackers and assorted teas. Using my portable sewing machine, she set up a mini-factory and began making postmaternity clothes for me and a snowsuit for Joseph. Having her there made it fun to be home and reduced the strain of new motherhood. Since she is a mother of six, an infant was not the strange and fearsome thing to her that it was to me.

Aside from the first night, the most difficult event of the first week was taking Joseph to get a bilirubin test. Newborns often develop jaundice because their immature livers cannot excrete all the bilirubin produced by the breakdown of excess red blood cells. If the bilirubin count goes too high, the infant may have to be placed under special lights to help the body absorb it.

I took Joseph to the lab. The lab technician had little experience with infants. I held him while she tried to extract what seemed to me a gallon of blood by repeatedly lancing his big toe and heel. When the technician turned to her trainee and asked if she would like to try, I said no. As it was, the procedure took forty-five minutes, and the technician had to squeeze out each drop. Joseph was screaming, and I felt as if she had squeezed all the blood out of me. I had to steel myself not to say aloud what I was thinking and to stay until the technician was finished.

The next day the doctor called to say the results showed the bilirubin count had gone up. We needed to have another test. I knew I could not go through that again, but I also knew Joseph had to have the test, so I took him to the hospital where the technicians frequently have to draw blood from babies. They took Joseph into another room and brought him back to me in fifteen minutes. It was a much less barbaric experience. This time his test results came back normal. Mom went with me both times and helped me keep my perspective—yes, he would live past the first week; no, he would not be psychologically damaged for the rest of his life by the experience.

Actually, Joseph has an easygoing personality so far. He cries to announce he is hungry or wet but does not have trouble with digestion or seem nervous.

March 3. He has fallen into a four-hour schedule, sleeping most of the time he is not eating, but awake and alert about two or three hours of the day. During that time we usually prop him up in his infant seat. Sometimes I give him a pacifier. From his throne he surveys his environment. He moves his blackish-blue globe-like eyes constantly. His mouth and hands are also in constant motion. My mother said, "He is very busy doing little things." He flexes his arms and hands, brings his hands to his mouth, purses his lips, makes sucking motions, frowns, smiles, stretches, cranes his neck, and lifts his arms up straight. All the while he is looking around. Sometimes he looks for a long time at something that appears insignificant to me, like the ceiling or the wall. He is enjoying merely using his eyes, although I know he cannot focus well yet.

I felt desolate yesterday afternoon when my mother left. Standing at the sink washing the dishes as she drove away, the whole weight of what had occurred suddenly came down on me. Without her, being a mother did not seem fun anymore, and I had to face my own ambivalence toward having an infant to care for. I could not lean on her positive attitude anymore.

I am afraid of Joseph. I am afraid he will have a need I can't meet, or that I will not be able to love him enough, or that he will manipulate me with his behavior. The truth is that I can meet Joseph's needs, even if I have to get advice from others to do it; that love grows and God is the source of an infinite supply of love; and finally, that I can trust his responses to be what they appear to be.

It will take a while for my confidence to grow. Each day I learn more about what this new person named Joseph is like and what his needs are. It has only been a week since he was born and less than a week since I brought him home. It is natural that I do not have mothering all figured out yet. In fact a large part of being a mother is learning. I enjoyed my child development courses, but this is the real thing, my own child. No course could prepare me for that.

I am gradually recovering my old shape. I am eight pounds away from my original weight, which means that, including the six pounds of fluids I gained the last two weeks of pregnancy, I have lost twenty-three pounds in a week. It feels good not to be pregnant, to be able to look at a pair of thin legs, to be able to see a waist again.

March 4. Today is my supposed due date and already I have had Joseph for over a week. This is the first full day I have been alone with him, and it has gone well. The things I learned from the nursery staff in the hospital have been invaluable. They showed me how to bathe Joseph, keeping him covered as much as possible where I am not washing. They told me about using a nonscented soap to avoid skin reactions and washing him only every other day. One nurse said that most of the products sold for babies are unnecessary expenditures. Their hair can be washed with soap twice a week, but should be combed every day to avoid cradlecap (flaking of the scalp). Vaseline is what nurses recommended for diaper rash. They showed me how to tuck him in snugly so that he feels secure. I usually put him in bed on his stomach so that his arms do not flail around, but he also likes to be on his side with a blanket rolled up behind him. Apparently it is not advisable to put newborns on their backs to sleep since they might spit up and choke.

In case Joseph is fussy the nurses told me to try patting his back, or changing his position, or burping him, or checking to see if he is wet, or giving him some water, or just holding him. They showed me how to hold Joseph with his head down and turned to the side if he chokes while drinking. One of the most valuable suggestions was how to deal with a baby when it starts being awake more. Wrap it in a receiving blanket and sit it in an infant seat covered with another blanket and give it a pacifier. Then the baby has a grandstand view of his world. Joseph likes that. He spends a couple of hours each day in his seat.

I grow in confidence as the days pass smoothly by. I am getting rest—and visitors continue to drop by, providing a pleasant distraction. The stitches are almost healed, and the uterine bleeding that followed delivery is lighter in color and less heavy today.

Motherhood is intense at first. There is no way around that. Every emotion is invested in the baby, whether I try to remain objective or not. I am trying to be aware of Tom's needs and the various other aspects of my life besides Joseph, but I am not very successful. My emotional energy is spent on Joseph, and there is little left for anything else. Striking a balance will take time.

The first thing Tom says when he comes home from work

is, "Has Joseph been asking for me?" He is fascinated by Joseph, but does not know quite what to do with him, since he is not big enough yet to toss up in the air and wrestle with.

Now that Joseph's schedule is more predictable, life is almost back to normal, with a difference. It has definitely been enriched.

> And I say
> "Oh for the wings of a dove
> to fly away and find rest."
> How far I would take my flight
> and make a new home in the desert!
> (Ps. 55:6-7)

Yesterday when things were going smoothly, I thought of life with a baby as being like a home in the desert. I am finding a new home, settling into a new way of life which is to a certain degree solitary, as a life in the desert would be. From a green, hilly land, where my time is my own, I go to a desert land. A desert has its advantages, though. It is the place where seekers have traditionally gone to find God. Jesus went to the desert for forty days before the beginning of his ministry in order to fast and pray.

It is difficult to build a home in the desert. There are few building materials; food and drink are scarce. There is intense heat in the day and cold at night. But the desert has a beauty all its own, and creatures it claims for its own. There is a desert spider called the sandtrap spider who catches its prey by digging a hole in the sand in such a way that a thin layer of sand is left covering it. The unwary insect crossing the pit, falls through and is devoured. I can adapt gracefully and be a survivor, or I can be a victim.

The heat of the desert is the intensity of learning to be a

93

mother and trying to do the right things. It is the heat that makes me turn to the Lord. I want to surrender more fully to God. What better way to do it than to serve this child at any hour of the day or night?

March 6. I do not agree with all Dr. Benjamin Spock says, but he makes an interesting point about the growth and development of an infant mirroring the development of the human race. In *Baby and Child Care*, he writes:

[They] start off in the womb as a single tiny cell, just as the first living thing appeared in the ocean. Weeks later, as they lie in the amniotic fluid in the womb, they have gills like fish. Toward the end of the first year of life, when they learn to clamber to their feet, they're celebrating that period millions of years ago when our ancestors got up off all fours. It's just at that time that babies are learning to use their fingers with skill and delicacy. Our ancestors stood up because they had found more useful things to do with their hands than walking on them.

The infant's development also mirrors our later spiritual development. At first the infant is totally self-absorbed, but as he gets older, he becomes more aware of his environment and interacts with it. He becomes better able to affect it and to manipulate it. Jesus tells us to go beyond our self-absorbed womb-like existence—far beyond—to deny ourselves in order to follow him and to serve our brothers and sisters. The temptation is to remain spiritual infants, concerned merely with our own needs. As always, the paradox of the gospel is present. Only by losing our lives in Christ will we find our true lives.

After a night of real frustration, I reread the psalmist's words about fleeing to the desert. They struck quite a different response in me this time. Joseph stayed up after his 6:00 P.M. feeding. He cried and could not go to sleep until 8:00 P.M. Then, when I fed him at 4:00 A.M., he would not go back to sleep until 5:00 A.M., though he was obviously tired. The incident was minor, but I was left emotionally spent. I couldn't understand Joseph. I didn't know whether to keep him up or not—I was so frustrated and tired. Then I thought with longing of a private desert. It could have rattlesnakes, spiders, scorching sand, but no babies.

The next day Joseph was back to normal. With a little rest, I could see light ahead and the black clouds passed.

It is presently 11:30 A.M. Joseph is sitting up in his seat with the sun pouring in the window. He has been awake for an hour contentedly peering around. I set two of his stuffed animals where he could easily see them and he has been carefully studying them. Their large, bright eyes catch his attention.

The more I hear about the difficulties other people have with their babies' sleeping and eating habits, the more I appreciate Joseph's calm disposition and (most of the time) good sleeping habits. We have discovered that he likes music. Often if he is restless, turning on a record calms him down. He seems especially fond of Mozart (such sophisticated tastes).

At Joseph's first checkup he weighed eight pounds five ounces. He has gained a pound in the week and two days since he came home from the hospital. The goal, according to the doctor, is one-half to one ounce per day. He has gained almost two ounces a day. I foresee big grocery bills. Already he has lost the red scrawny newborn look.

March 7. I have not experienced what is classically called postpartum depression, but I tend to be weepy when Tom comes home in the evening, especially if I'm tired. I want to get out of the house now. In the two weeks since I came home from the hospital, I've been out a total of about three hours without Joseph.

If someone asked me how I feel as a new mother, I would have to answer: profoundly ignorant. My question at the moment is how long to let Joseph stay up in the evening after eating. He seems to go to sleep less quickly after each feeding than he did at first, but I have found that sometimes I can put him in his cradle before he is asleep with a toy to look at, and he will fall gradually asleep. When he is overtired or overstimulated, he cries, and rocking him only makes things worse. Tom gets on edge and says, "Why can't you do something?" I become increasingly tense and irritated. Finally Joseph and I exhaust each other, and he falls asleep.

I wait impatiently for the weather to get warmer so we can go out. I hardly remember what the sun feels like anymore. Winter is exile. I love the smells and sounds and warmth of spring and summer.

March 9.   I went for a walk and a visit to the bookstore by myself today. Yesterday's heavy snow is melting in today's mild temperature. The streets are running with water, and a big patch of snow fell on my shoulder as I walked under an awning. The weather cannot make up its mind whether to hold onto winter or to give way to spring.

In the bookstore I noticed the woman at the counter looking at me, and I wondered what she saw. I was wearing a wraparound skirt my sister made for me that I have not had time to shorten, plus an old coat that ties at the waist and probably shows the extra poundage I am carrying around. I wondered, though, if my new interior state showed. Could she see that I am now a mother? Could she see my dignity? Could she see my maturity? I feel like a different person. Years seem to have passed by due to the new weight of responsibility.

Although it is difficult to maintain a sense of humor, and I feel ignorant and trapped at times, I am happy. Becoming a mother has been less of an adjustment than becoming a wife. That required a major alteration in self-image. This is more of an augmentation and enrichment of the life Tom and I have already established together.

March 11. Tonight my younger sister Agnes arrives from Washington. We're getting more visitors from my family now that there is the enticement of a baby.

My family was a haven for growing up. I can think of no better preparation for having my own than the one I grew up in.

The years I remember best were at our house on Rosemary Street in North Carolina. We lived in a five-bedroom clapboard house near town with an expansive front- and backyard dotted with old oak and walnut trees. My parents did extensive work on it to make it suitable for six active children and all their pets. They added a glassed-in sun porch, took out the wall between the dining room and living room to leave an old brick fireplace standing between the two rooms, and added a wooden deck.

In the evenings my parents often entertained friends from the university where my father taught English, but we rarely had overnight guests.

We grew up in the South in years that were turbulent with racial change, but the climate in that world was hopeful. There was hope that prejudice could be changed, that the poor could be educated, and that eventually poverty itself would cease to exist. In general there was a feeling that the world was moving ahead toward a better future. My parents marched and picketed segregated shops in town, while at home we children collected June bugs and lightning bugs in jars and played Capture the Flag until it was too dark to see anymore. We made pets of caterpillars by tying strings around their necks; we danced to a record called "The Elephant Stomp"; and we played in the rain in our bathing suits. We enjoyed life.

Now the future does not look so bright. Energy shortages, worldwide political unrest, and proliferation of nuclear weapons make things look bleak. What about Joseph? What kind of a life will he live? Can we give him a childhood free of fear? I can only have faith. I believe—I must believe—that life is a gift at any cost.

I learned a great deal from my parents about parenting. They made mistakes. They argued on occasion. Like most parents, they expected too much sometimes. But when I add up my experience of childhood, the good far outweighs the bad.

My mother was thoroughly committed to us, self-sacrificing and loving. She spent time with us, and she was there when we needed her. She was highly intelligent, encouraged our endeavors, nurtured our creativity, stimulated us with books and concerts and lessons, and refused to let us settle for the second-rate.

My father was just as committed to us, though he gave of himself in different ways. He was a good disciplinarian; he told us stories, read us books, made a puppet theater for us, devised treasure hunts with rhyming clues for our birthday parties, played on the floor with us, and took us on trips to pick berries.

Even if I listed all their attributes and qualities, I would be far from putting my finger on how my parents affect my behavior as a parent, because I have been influenced not only in countless ways by them, but also by other things in my environment. Much of what I learned from my parents about parenting is probably subconscious. The threads become too entangled to unravel, but I am glad for the life I had while growing up.

There are many stages to parenting. The parenting my parents gave us in early childhood was different from what they gave in adolescence, and the parenting in early adulthood different still. They are still parenting now that I am twenty-six and a parent myself. We never get over needing our parents, especially their support and encouragement, even though we grow beyond depending on them and basing our decisions on their desires.

March 13. Joseph has switched to a three-hour schedule during the day and four at night. He is growing fast. Already his hands and fingernails look bigger, and he is filling out his clothes. He smiles after eating, but not in response to anyone yet. He can squirm to the corner of his cradle. He watches objects close to him for long periods of time. In the past few days he has developed an angry cry and look. When he knows I am about to feed him, but haven't yet, he lets out a wail and scowls at me.

He can find his thumb easily when he wants to suck it. When awake he is happy to look around for about an hour. After that he starts fidgeting and trying to put his hands in his mouth. Then he needs to eat or go to sleep again.

Last night we took him with us to a meeting. He had been up about an hour and handled a lot by Tom and my sister. He was obviously tense and overtired, but couldn't relax. Tom and I in turn became very tense and when Joseph kept fussing, I finally left the hall and took him where he could cry without disturbing anyone. Then he fell into a deep sleep and slept four hours. I collapsed when we got home. I cried myself and felt exhausted. Today I am still tired, but I can understand better what happened. I now put him in bed after an hour of being up instead of waiting for him to fall asleep.

March 14. Letting Joseph cry for a little while before going to sleep seems to be working well. I don't know if he will have to cry every time before he goes to sleep or if I will find other ways of helping him go to sleep.

The book I am reading says a "very active baby will wriggle up to the corner of his crib by the time he is three or four weeks old." Joseph did that the first night he was home from the hospital. It also says "some strong month-old babies will lift their heads off the sheet when lying on their stomachs." He does that now at three weeks. Obviously, a superior child (and a biased mother).

In the first seven days of life, the book goes on to say, most newborns spend four-fifths of their time sleeping. They usually eat every three hours. Joseph slept when he was not eating, but he only ate every four hours. Now he has gone to three.

When they are born, infants cannot adapt to bright lights but that improves within twenty-four hours. It was pitiful to see Joseph after he was born trying to keep his eyes closed under the bright lights of the delivery room. In the nursery the bright lights stay on continually. When out of the lights, Joseph opened his eyes and looked around with great alertness. The focus of the eye is about seven and a half inches at birth. Objects closer or farther away are blurred.

Researchers have found that infants stare at a patterned suface longer than at a plain surface and prefer a human face to any other sight. They like things that move and are about eight to ten inches away. I have found that Joseph will stare for a long time at stuffed animals that have faces with big eyes. He also likes to look at the night light in his room. He has a hard time focusing on our faces for long periods perhaps because they move in and out of focus so often. His eyes still cross at times and are not perfectly coordinated. They were black when he was born, but are getting bigger and bluer as he gets older.

I have been afraid of overstimulating Joseph by holding him a lot. I thought too much holding would keep him from sleeping. I now read that stimulation up to a point is good for babies. They need it and in fact cry less and are healthier when stimulated. That doesn't mean I should play with Joseph all the time he is awake, but I shouldn't leave him alone the whole time either.

In the first year, an infant increases his length by a third and triples his weight. No wonder Joseph sleeps so much, if he is growing at that rate. He probably weighs about nine pounds now and getting big round cheeks.

March 16. No writing this weekend, I spent all my time with Tom and the baby.

Last weekend I was continually frustrated because I had a way of handling Joseph that worked out and Tom handled him differently. I didn't want to keep telling Tom how to do things, but I didn't want him to keep Joseph awake too long or overstimulate him. This weekend we were both more relaxed, although Saturday morning started out with some difficulty.

I was up a number of times Friday night. Joseph demanded to be fed every three hours that night. On Saturday morning he started at 7:30. After I fed him he stayed awake. At 9:00 I went to the grocery store; Tom assured me he could rock Joseph to sleep. When I returned at 10:30, Tom was frenzied. Apparently Joseph went to sleep for a little while, then woke up about half an hour before I got back, hungry and crying, even though his normal feeding time wasn't until 11:00. After I fed him and got him to sleep, I felt worn out. Then Tom's mother called to say she was coming over to see Joseph. I was so tired that I took a nap and got up about half an hour after she arrived.

We had been invited out for dinner at a friend's house, but the friend called to say she had a bad cold, so we didn't go. Instead Tom and I had a nice dinner and talk, which greatly refreshed me. I needed the refreshment because after I gave Joseph his evening feeding he wouldn't or couldn't relax and stayed awake until about 8:30 with loud crying and apparent discomfort. Finally, when nothing else worked, we put him in bed, and he cried himself to sleep within ten minutes. It is hard to let him do that, but he seems to need it. I think he is sensitive to overhandling and tension around him. The evening is regularly a hard time for him. I am trying a few things. I am cutting down on the coffee I drink to see if this affects Joseph's behavior after nursing, and I am borrowing a swing and mobile from a friend. It's easy for me to feel that if only I were more experienced I would know what to do, but I am finding that everyone's baby is different. It is hard to beat trial and error.

Saturday night he was again on a three hour schedule and I got minimal sleep. I gave him a bath Sunday morning, which relaxed him. He then slept heavily for four hours. Tom and I took turns going to church. We had a meeting at 4:30, and I kept worrying about Joseph's being fussy. He fell asleep in his carrier and slept until we got home at 7:30. Then he began the pattern of crying and tenseness once again. When all else had failed I fed him again. Then he went to sleep, woke and cried at 9:30, and didn't wake up again until 1:30, then again at 5:15. A much better schedule for me. I rested this morning. Tom brought him to me at 5:30—all changed, calm, and ready to eat.

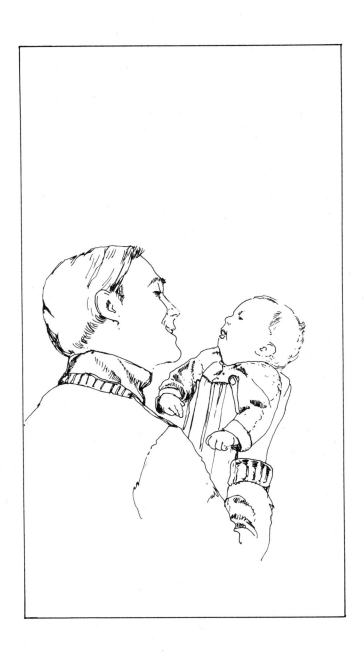

Tom is handling Joseph well. He thrives on the fatherhood but is frustrated when he doesn't know how to quiet Joseph or thinks Joseph is not responding to him. It is wonderful to see the father developing in Tom.

I think I am adjusting well to motherhood. The difficult times have been when I haven't been able to get enough sleep or when Joseph has been fussy for no reason. Without this journal the adjustment might have been harder. It is an outlet for me. While I am writing and doing research for it, the need for other outlets diminishes.

March 19. There is so much joy in life if we can only experience it. Too often we focus on the negative parts of our experience while ignoring the positive. I have found this especially true in having a baby. People ask me how I like staying at home, expecting that I will say I am bored. Some mothers complain that children require great sacrifices, that they are sick of being stuck at home, that this child or that is sick again, that they wish they had a job, that they are tired. It is *too rare* to hear a mother expressing delight in her children. The negative is contagious, but the positive can be equally contagious.

Children pick up their parents' attitude toward them. This attitude can affect their self-image as they grow older. Parents can point out the good and reinforce their children's self-image, or they can focus on the negative and contribute to poor self-image.

All this is not to say everything about parenting is rosy. Everyone feels tired and has bad days. But a basically positive attitude can put all of those minor problems in their proper perspective.

I was struck today as I was reading the Gospel of Mark by Jesus' words to the parents of the child who had died and was raised by Jesus from the dead. When the parents told

Jesus not to bother coming because the child was already dead, he said, "Do not be afraid, only have faith" (5:37). Belief replaces fear. The story reminded me of the fears I had about having a baby and how I needed to practice faith. Now I see that those fears were groundless, as are most of our fears.

March 24. Joseph was four weeks old last Friday. He is fun to play with. Today he smiled a full smile, looking straight at me. He is not frowning as much as he did at first and is happy during the time he is awake. Strangely enough, his schedule is getting less regular. I would have thought it would become more regular. Sometimes he goes two hours between feedings, sometimes three, or four. It is very unpredictable. At night he sometimes sleeps up to five hours, sometimes only three. He has been waking up sooner in between feedings during the day. I don't know if he is hungry or just not sleepy. He might not know either.

I have been trying to write for two hours. Every time I sit down to write, Joseph starts crying. I am on call. Now he is in bed, but I can still hear him making little sounds in the other room.

He is making his first social noises. When he is contented he makes low hoarse sounds from the back of his throat. Today I noticed two other new things. He grasped his own hand, and he looked at it when it came before his eyes. His movements are becoming more controlled. He does not startle and throw his arms out when I change him. He does, however, regularly manage to wet himself and any person unlucky enough to be standing nearby when he is being changed.

I have started running again. It feels grand. It is a good way of releasing tension and getting a change of scenery. I must find a way of doing this every day. Perhaps I can find someone who also has a baby who would like to go to the track with me. Then we could take turns watching the babies and running. Or I could try to fit the running in before dinner.

How soon do infants recognize their parents? I have noticed a difference in the way Joseph responds to me and the way he responds to other people. He smiles three or four times a day at me and, if fussing, will quiet down when I hold him. He watches me when I am in the room and looks at me when I am talking. I notice him doing that more with me than with Tom.

The books say that as early as four months of age a baby can differentiate between its mother and other people. It smiles and vocalizes more in her presence and follows her with its eyes. A month after a baby first shows this attachment behavior toward its mother, it begins showing it toward other members of the family. Most babies show attachment behavior toward other members of the family within a couple of months after showing it toward their mothers. As might be expected, sensitivity to the infant's signals and the amount and nature of interaction between mother and infant are the most important factors in attachment developing.

March 31. Joseph is growing more predictable. Maybe Joseph feels my sense of contentment. He is doing several new things. He likes to stand on my lap supported by my hands. He pulls at his mouth with his fingers, and he is becoming increasingly sociable. In fact he is progressively less willing to entertain himself. He wants to be held and played with. Not too much of a problem, because he is so much fun to play with.

He weighs almost eleven pounds now. That is the weight at which the books say he should begin to sleep through the night. I do not expect it to happen right away. His 2:00 A.M. and 5:00 or 6:00 A.M. schedule of waking is too consistent. Rarely does he go beyond five hours between feedings. The norm is three to four. It is not that difficult to get up anyway. Last night went by fast. When he woke up at 5:30, I groaned because I thought it was 3:30.

Friday night we took Joseph with us to Tom's boss's house for dinner. Joseph was fine until I put him to bed upstairs in his car bed. He slept briefly, then woke up crying and continued to cry all evening. He knew, even at his age, that he was in a strange house and a strange bed.

April

Each day brings more changes. Joseph has a rash on his face. It started when he was about four weeks old as red spots on his face and neck. It became more pronounced when he was hot or upset. This type of rash is common between the fourth and tenth week. It is a reaction to the hormones in the mother's milk and the result of skin pores opening up. I noticed one of his breasts is slightly swollen—also a normal reaction to the hormones in my milk.

I was given a foam rubber molded cushion to put in the bathtub when I give Joseph a bath. I thought he would enjoy being in the water rather than having sponge baths, but he screamed every time I put him in to the point of becoming hysterical. Perhaps he does not like being undressed and having his limbs unrestrained. I tried putting him in the water wrapped in a receiving blanket. That worked very well. He only cried briefly. Once in the water, I unwrapped him and washed him. It is a bother to hang the blankets around to dry, but avoiding the hysterics is worth it.

I also started feeding him before bathing him. The nurses at the hospital recommended not feeding until after the bath so he would not spit up if he got upset by the water. The problem is that he cries lustily for his dinner and will consider nothing else until he is fed.

A leap forward today! Joseph started batting at the ring of multicolored keys I hung on the side of his cradle. He stared at them and then moved his hand toward them and pushed them. Then he did it over and over again. That takes a lot of coordination. It means he can move his hand consciously toward an object that his eyes see.

April 3.   Today is Holy Thursday in the church calendar. This past week has been dreary. The sky is like gray granite.

Holy Thursday, a day of preparation for Good Friday. Jesus washing the feet of his disciples. Community: washing the feet of our brothers and sisters and letting our feet be washed. The latter is sometimes more difficult, and it says something important about the truth of our relationships. There was a reason for Jesus insisting that the disciples let him wash their feet. First, it was an example of how they were to act and a concrete example of the fact that Jesus came to serve. Also, letting someone serve is displaying trust in that person. It means giving up a certain prideful independence, and trusting that the person who is serving will not take advantage of the situation by later insisting on the debt owed. It is believing in that person's love, not believing he resents what he is doing. Basically, it is allowing ourselves to be in relationship with another. Trust (giving up independence based on pride) and letting ourselves be in relationship with others are essential for the existence of a true community.

It is difficult to serve sometimes. I find myself thinking I could be doing more than folding clothes, vacuuming, washing dishes, and taking care of a baby. It is humbling to do the menial tasks. The truth is that I could be doing other things, but this is where I am right now. These are the opportunities I have to serve. These are the tasks I am challenged to do well, not some imagined others that I might choose for myself. Let me do them gladly.

April 7.   The rain is pattering outside, and I have turned the lights on. The combination of the rain and the lamps creates a cozy atmosphere. It is the right day for a crackling fire and a good book. Outside I hear a bird chirping in the rain. He doesn't mind the water dripping on him. He and his buddies are enjoying their bath.

I can get lost in baby care and all the minutiae of running a house. I noticed last night when we went over to a friend's house for dinner that I was perfectly content to sit quietly and not engage in the discussion. The orbit of life draws in with a baby. I am absorbed within the small circle of husband and child and tempted to lose myself there. For once the forces vying inside me are quiet. I am becalmed.

Yesterday I took Joseph for his six weeks checkup. He weighs eleven pounds, five ounces and is twenty-two and a half inches long. Both measurements are just above the fiftieth percentile for his age. In other words, he is pretty normal.

The bad news is that his bilirubin is still higher than it should be. The doctor said it is probably due to the breast milk. He wanted to be sure, so for two days I have to feed Joseph formula. Then he will be tested again. If the results show significantly less jaundice, the doctor will know the jaundice is caused by the milk, but I can go on breast feeding and the jaundice will gradually disappear. If it is not the milk, he will have to do further tests.

All this is very inconvenient. The breast is a wonderful invention. No bottles, no formula, no expense. I am inundated now with the paraphernalia of bottle feeding. Last night I took a bottle of formula out of the refrigerator for Joseph's 2:00 A.M. feeding and gave it to him without warming it up. I thought that since the doctor said he could drink cold water, he could drink cold formula, too. Definitely not true. I fed him the whole bottle, and he promptly spit up the whole bottle, all over me, himself, and the floor. After that he was wide awake for another hour, but would not eat anymore, even when I heated it. I was a tragic picture. My bathrobe was streaked with regurgitated formula, and my pajamas were soaking wet from the milk dripping from my breasts.

I borrowed a breast pump, because without some way of

draining off the extra milk, the breasts become sore and engorged. The pump is a slightly glorified bicycle horn. There is a bulb at one end and a horn at the other. The horn is supposed to fit over the breast while the bulb suctions out the milk. In theory.

I sat for half an hour in the bathroom feeling foolish, attempting to extract milk with the pump. Drop by slow drop it came. At the end of thirty minutes I had just covered the bottom of the attached bottle with a thin whitish fluid and my breasts were becoming increasingly sore.

Finally I gave up and started squeezing the milk out by hand into a cup. In another half an hour I had half a cup and was wet all over. What a temptation it was to say the heck with it and sneak in to let Joseph extract the milk for me. The mouth of a baby is perfectly designed for that and there is no good substitute. At 4 A.M. I was up again standing under the kitchen light wearily squeezing out milk.

These two days seem like ten. I have been so busy that I have hardly seen a glimpse of Tom. My idea of togetherness is not sitting side-by-side in bed while I try to pump milk into a cup. Tomorrow morning it will be over.

I have made some interesting discoveries from all this. One, that when I am not breast feeding Joseph, I miss the sense of oneness with him that it gives me. Two, that breast feeding takes longer than bottle feeding. That appears to be a disadvantage, but actually the time spent in feeding is a good time to be together. On the side of bottle feeding, Joseph sleeps longer on formula. It is heavier than breast milk.

April 10. Another cold gray day, but there are overtures of spring, so I will forgive the weather. Today I saw, amid the old leaves and fallen fence behind the house, the courageous white blossoms of a hyacinth. I have been staying inside, defeated by the weather, but this afternoon I am going to fight back and take Joseph for a walk.

I had my six weeks checkup yesterday. I have recovered completely from the birth, the doctor said. Because I stopped breast feeding for two days, my period started. The body is so sensitive. Even two days was enough for everything to start changing gears. I also almost stopped producing milk.

Joseph is becoming increasingly attached to me. It is a pleasurable as well as a frightening experience. More than ever I am not independent. But love gives without counting the cost.

I am losing my autonomy in other ways, too. Being at home is certainly different from working. I have to plan my day around Joseph's schedule now. When I was working coming home meant being free to do whatever I wanted. Now home is where I am on call.

A friend pointed out that I implicitly said yes to this when I got married. Having a child and being responsible for it is a further spelling out of that yes. It is the echo of Jesus' yes to his father. The reverberations are like the tremors of an earthquake that shake and reorder every item in the house. Like most people I would rather avoid the total yes, the total surrender.

Lately I have experienced a recurrent fear of God, his authority, and the cost of following him. Dietrich Bonhoeffer and many other modern Christians were willing to die for their faith. Would I be willing to do that? Some days I do not bother to pray. What is faith worth to me? Would I risk my life for it? Can I even surrender to God this everyday existence?

I watched a six-month-old baby last night. How sophisticated she was. She smiled at everyone. She looked at the pictures in a book by herself and pointed at things on

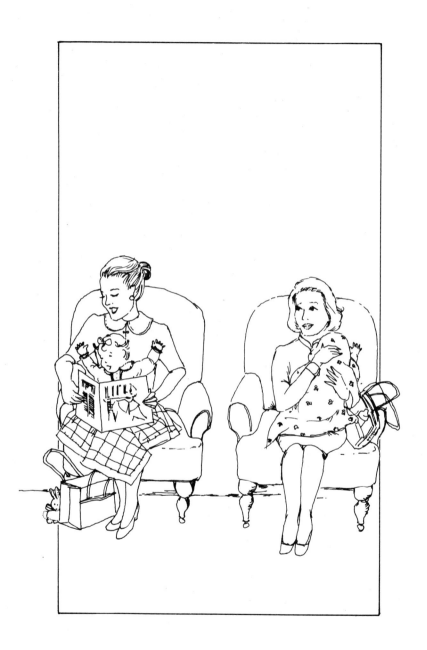

the pages. She passed the book from one hand to the other and searched for her mother's hand under the blanket when it was hidden. Seeing her made me look forward to Joseph at that age.

April 14. I am very tired. We had Joseph baptized yesterday. All day Saturday I cooked for the reception. On Sunday morning I finished the cooking and got Joseph ready. He was fussy all weekend, probably because my milk supply is still not back to normal.

The ceremony was disappointing to me because I was trying to keep Joseph from crying. As soon as the ceremony started, he decided he wanted dinner. Then, when I expected him to cry he didn't. When I wash his hair he usually wails, but when the priest poured water on his head for the baptism, Joseph opened his eyes wide and smiled.

April 15. It is snowing!

The scratchy squeaks of birds calling
    like rusty wheels turning,
    sound from amid the snowflakes.
Are they brave hearts or foolish?
Will their sounds fall frozen and hungry from the sky
    or will those who hope soon spread their wings
    and come back leading in the sun?

Yesterday Tom brought me some daisies. He noticed that I have been feeling depressed and is trying to make me feel better. A combination of factors have gotten me down. One of the biggest is the physical adjustment after pregnancy. My body has gone through so many changes that my self-image is affected. I question whether I am still attractive with the extra pounds I still have to get rid of. The doctor says I may not lose those until I stop breast feeding. I question my basic femininity. Without realizing it, I have been infected with the media's ideals of the figure-perfect American woman.

It is also hard to adjust to the demands of breast feeding. I am tired during the day and am still getting up during the night for feedings. Perhaps what affects me most is hormonal changes. I notice that my face is oily after being dry for much of the pregnancy.

This morning I walked to a friend's house with Joseph in the front carrier. I enjoyed getting out, but I am still not myself. The responsibility of a baby weighs heavily on me today.

I expected the adjustments of motherhood to pass in seven weeks, but perhaps that is unrealistic. As I settle into a routine, the full meaning of the change is coming home to me. There are days when I check to see if I've worn a path from living room to kitchen to bedroom. I get tired of looking at the familiar.

April 16. Finally—sun. The birds were right after all—there is reason for hope. The two evergreens beside the steps are sending out new green branches. They were brutally clipped by our landlord two years ago, and we thought they had died. The lilac that looks naked and spindly in the winter is now twinkling with green buds on the ends of each branch. When the sun comes out I begin to think of our patch of grass as a yard again and of our patch of dirt as a garden. We have daisies and alyssum, plus an overabundance of chives and parsley in the garden.

I am more interested in growing something nonutilitarian like flowers than I am in growing vegetables. So much of my life is spent in pursuing practical ends that it is a luxury to spend time on something that makes life richer. From the looks of creation, God thought beauty was at least as important as utility.

A bird is taking a dust bath next door, leaning over and rubbing his chest in the dust, then fluttering his wings. He looks like he is enjoying himself. Such a small thing, but he takes pleasure in it. Now there is a throng of birds chattering and playing in the dirt.

Pleasure can come from very simple things, like looking around the dinner table at my family. Tom and I can sit for an hour watching Joseph make faces and play, and he is our entertainment. I had thought it would be hard to sit and play with a baby as parents do, but I was wrong. He gives us pleasure, and we give him pleasure.

One of the worst results of materialism is losing sight of the real sources of joy: the people, the things we do together (flying a kite, playing cards, cooking out, reading quietly together in the same room).

One vivid memory I have from childhood is of lying on the warm stones of our walkway with the sun heating me to the bone watching the ants going about their business. I was spying on another world. I am grateful for the time during that growing up period that allowed me to lie there. Times like that made me feel strongly how important it is to see, notice, and enjoy what is around one every day. Our lives are not long. Already a third of mine has passed. I want it to have quality regardless of the quantity.

April 17.   Today I took Joseph for a walk in the front carrier. It was so warm that I didn't have to cover his head. At first he squinted and was bothered by the breeze on his face. Then he got used to being outside and peered intently around as we walked.

We saw a woman in a store who had a baby in the same type of carrier. Babies are a natural introduction to people.

116

We had a talk about our babies' behavior at different ages. Another woman stopped me on the street to ask whether he was a boy or girl and then kissed him. The same reaction at the grocery store. An older woman could not keep her eyes off Joseph and told me the whole story of her family while we waited in line.

My milk supply is back to normal now and Joseph is sleeping better, usually going three to four hours between feedings. He has also rediscovered his thumb. All of a sudden he realized he could suck his thumb instead of crying when he was put to bed. He lies quietly now until he falls asleep and, if he wakes up too soon, will suck his thumb and go back to sleep. Yesterday he slept so much that I started missing him. He still does not sleep through the night, but before I had him I never knew there was a point during the first year when children do normally sleep through. If he does sleep through the night during the next few months it will seem like a bonus.

April 18.   A rough day and it is only half over. This morning I leaned over to pop the toast out of the toaster while I was holding Joseph and his hand touched the toaster. He was burned slightly on two fingers. The doctor wrapped them in gauze to protect against infection. The results from his blood test last week came back and showed that his bilirubin still has not gone down as it should have after stopping the breast milk for two days. Now he has to have another blood test on Monday. The high bilirubin might be something hereditary related to the fact that Tom has consistently had a high liver enzyme. Joseph is taking it quite nonchalantly, eating and sleeping up a storm.

We have been out for walks almost every day. To Joseph everything is new. He cranes his neck to look around. He

117

doesn't know how to breathe when a breeze comes, so he sniffs in.

April 22. Joseph and I are out on the porch. He is in an automatic swing and is not fussing. The last couple of days he has wanted me to pick him up every time I put him down and has been eating every two hours. The reason yesterday was clear. In the morning I had to take him for blood test. He had to be stuck in the heel six or seven times to get the blood they needed. He was upset all day after that. He cried easily, wanted to be held, and couldn't fall asleep for a long time in the evening. When we put him to bed at eight, he was obviously tired, but kept crying and crying, so we put him in the swing to calm him down. Finally he went to sleep.

Today I talked to a nurse about the ten pounds I still have to lose. She said the body builds up a store of fat during pregnancy so that I can have reserves to draw from when the baby is nursing. That reserve is used up after the first three or four months, so after that there should be no problem losing weight. I have another month before I should be concerned.

I am tired right now. I have dark circles under my eyes, but I am happy.

I am trying to stay home as much as possible this week because Joseph has been so uncomfortable. Regularity of environment should help him settle down.

April 25. The word *marvel* has been coming to mind lately in regard to the experience of having a child and, on a broader scale, to life itself. Knowing there is a creator broadens my sense of life's wonder. Life is not a happy (or some might say unhappy) accident. It is the gift of a loving God.

In Isaiah 44:24, speaking to Israel, God says it was he "who made you, who formed you from the womb."

Scientific discoveries enhance the miraculous nature of life. How many millions of combinations of genes are possible, yet this one came to be. This me. This self. This child of mine. This Joseph.

It increases my wonder to see the multitude of forms creation has taken. What kind of God is it that thought of elephants as well as organisms so small that their existence must be guessed at, mosses and grasses as well as redwood trees, deserts as well as oceans? Human beings have been occupied with the study of God's creation as long as he has existed and still scientists shake their heads at the vast amount they do not know.

Each creature has its own story. Volumes have been written on the behavior of honey bees. Researchers are just beginning to understand how it is that various migratory animals return to predetermined locations year after year, some of them without having made the journey previously. As large as a whale or as fragile as a butterfly, pushed on by an overwhelming urge, they travel thousands of miles to reach their goals.

I wonder at the change of seasons: how relentless it is, how grateful I always am for each change, how our natures seem to need change, how even our own lives operate on a seasonal basis. The measure of how well we are adjusted to life is the measure of how well we can adapt to the new seasons in our lives.

I wonder at where I fit into all this. I am part of creation. I am inextricably bound up in life and involved in processes like childbirth that I feel I have little to do with. Life goes on around and in me. I am aware, though, that my spirit (my self) is something different. It is in this world now, but will not always be. It is attached to this life, but will be part of a life to come. It is a part of creation that is special. Once created it does not succumb to the processes of aging and deterioration that affect other parts of creation. It is meant to become a thing more and more glorious as the years go by, actually reflecting God's glory.

> And we, with our unveiled faces reflecting like mirrors the brightness of the Lord, all grow brighter and brighter as we are turned into the image that we reflect; this is the work of the Lord who is Spirit.
>
> (II Cor. 3:18)

Later in the same letter Paul writes:

> Though this outer man of ours may be falling into decay, the inner man is renewed day by day. Yes, the troubles which are soon over, though they weigh little, train us for the carrying of a weight of eternal glory which is out of all proportion to them.
>
> (II Cor. 4:16b-18)

We are "bound for glory." When Jesus became man he was showing us what path our life should take. We are born into a world turned away from God, sharers in a communal guilt from the offenses of mankind. At baptism we are washed clean of that guilt by the power of Christ's death and resurrection, the act by which he took our place in paying for our sins. We enter into the kingdom of God, we declare ourselves for him and not for his enemy. Then we follow him; we try to do the will of the Father, as Jesus did in his life. At the end we must die as other members of creation do, but that which is incorruptible follows Jesus to the resurrection and is freed to live fully in God's presence—something mortal man can never achieve for himself.

It is so good, the plan is so immense and all-encompassing, that it is hard to grasp and hard to believe. Why is it easier to believe something bad than something good? Is it the fallen side of our nature tugging at us? Perhaps it is because when we have looked to men for things in the past we have been disappointed and to avoid another disappointment we would rather not hope. Yet hope is a taste of God. It is the flavor of his presence. We cannot experience God and not hope.

April 26. When I look at this mystery of the gospel, it is like turning a gem in my hand. At times it appears lucid and clear; at times it is murky and hard to comprehend—but it is always fascinating. It is as if the light shining through that stone were the only light illuminating the world.

A passage in the psalms reads, "By your light we see the light" (36:9). It is a phrase I ponder. I like to think it means that God is the pure light, the pure beauty, the pure goodness. All around us and in one another there are elements of light and darkness. The light is mixed and diffused. By contemplating the pure light we begin to recognize it around us and see God in one another. That is why knowing God makes the world more marvelous. We may experience the world as not estranged from ourselves. Nature and people around us manifest to one degree or another the God that we know.

April 28. This morning I am taking Joseph back to the doctor's office. His last blood tests showed that he has one liver enzyme a little higher than normal—a condition which Tom has also. Today he has to have more blood drawn for another test, plus his first shot. I don't know whether it is harder for him or for me. I hate to see him continually poked with needles.

I found out yesterday that the baby of one of the couples in our Lamaze class died at two months of crib death. Knowing how much we love Joseph already at just over two months old, I knew what anguish that couple must be going through. They must be asking why and are probably angry at God. I wish I knew the answer, but the question goes deeper. Why do we live in a world subject to death at all? Why do tragedies happen to innocent people?

Until Christ comes again we are still subject to the powers of evil at war with God. Until the Gospel has been preached to every nation and the present age has ripened to its conclusion, we are in the midst of spiritual combat. Senseless tragedies occur. I do know, though, that as that child was with God in his mind from the moment of creation, it has never left him and is with him now. I cannot wait until we are with God face-to-face and all the questions are answered, sorrows healed, pains assuaged, and our spirits filled with joy.

Spring

Joseph is like the lilac tree beside the house. Each day it is fuller with its load of new green leaves and purple buds. Each day Joseph's personality becomes more evident and new achievements are added to his repertoire.

I am useless when he is awake. I do nothing but sit and watch him or play with him. In the morning he is very happy. He fires a barrage of smiles up at me as I am changing him and smiles to himself while sitting in his chair or playing.

His newest discovery is his hands. About five days ago he started noticing his feet but only yesterday did he start looking at his hands. Sucking his thumb might have made him more aware of his hands. At any rate he can entertain himself for long periods of time just by examining them.

He still keeps his fists closed most of the time. He brings his arm up and twists his hand around from the wrist to look at as if it were some magnificent work of art. His arm movements are undulating and graceful, like a snake moving to the snake charmer's music, although he sometimes bumps his hand against his face when it comes too close.

While he was playing with his hands today, he kept drawing up his legs and twisting his body as if he were trying to turn over. Soon he will be able to.

As he becomes more aware of his environment, it is harder to put him to sleep anywhere other than in his own bed. He just cries. Other mothers assure me this phase does not last long. I hope not because it makes going out anywhere difficult.

About seven months ago I sensed God telling me that I needed to have more faith that the future would be good, and I needed to be more thankful for my present circumstances. I was at a low point then. I was pregnant and feeling more and more circumscribed. Since then I have prayed often for a change of heart. I have repented of not trusting God, and I have looked around me for things to be thankful for.

I can see a definite change in my attitude toward life. I can accept the need to go gladly into what is ahead for me, embracing it fully, the suffering as well as the good, and to be ready to serve. I now understand that I resented the kind of life I felt Tom was leading me towards.

I feel freer now than I have for a long time and look forward to the future. It is a challenge to go forward gladly, but also exciting. It is as if I had been waiting a long time to start on a hard march. Finally the news comes to begin, news I have been dreading, but once I start I want to run. It is a relief to begin the next stage in my life. The reality is much easier than my imaginings. And for Christians, there is one who goes before to prepare the way, one who strengthens us at each turn.

May 7.   Today we took Joseph to the liver clinic. They decided not to pursue his case any further. Joseph has a high enzyme count like Tom's, but Tom's has probably been high all his life and has never caused any problems. Joseph has a clean bill of health.

May 15.   We had babysitters last night and the night before. Joseph slept both nights from the time we left at 7:45 until I woke him up to eat at 10:30. I feel freer now that I can leave him for an evening. After I feed him before going to bed myself, he sleeps until six or seven o'clock in the morning.

I am experiencing a feeling when I am with Tom and Joseph such as I only experienced before while growing up in my own family: a naturalness and familiarity, and an instinctive knowing of one another.

This morning after feeding Joseph I gave him a bath in his dishpan bathtub in the kitchen sink. He prefers it to the regular bathtub because he can sit up in it and it is not so big. He no longer cries when I wash his hair and put him in the water. Instead, a look of pleasure appears on his face, and he will stay in as long as I let him. He likes to lift his feet out of the water to look at them and splash with them.

He is more interested in toys, especially ones that make a sound when he moves them. I disapproved of parents buying their children large numbers of toys, but I can understand now how it happens.

May 16. Joseph is constantly exploring with his hands and watching them, even while he is nursing. He touches my shirt with his little finger, then with the rest of his fingers. All the time his eyes are wide open watching his hand. Next I see that he has noticed my navy blue jacket, but it is going to be harder to reach. He throws his arm up so that his hand will land close to the jacket. Finally he is able to touch the jacket. Every few minutes his eyes go to my face for an instant, as if checking to make sure I am still there.

The big plant on the table next to where I nurse him is more interesting to him than the mobile we put up. When I move him close to it, he bats the leaves. He is working on bringing his thumb and forefinger together, but for now it is an accomplishment when he can grasp something with his whole hand. Soon he will be grabbing everything in sight.

May 22. It is time to draw these reflections to a conclusion. Joseph is three months old today. I have not reached an ending; rather I have made a beginning in this process of being a mother and wife. My nine-months journey and beyond has been an exciting and sometimes frightening adventure, full of new experiences.

I am enjoying this time in my life, but I enjoyed other times also. The goal is not marriage or motherhood. The goal is a life alive in the Holy Spirit, regardless of our state in life. The Spirit gives richness and substance to the present.

I hear the birds making raucous noises outside. They were right to hope for spring. This spring has been a time of reaping, a time to be thankful. We mourn enough when it is time for mourning. Let us rejoice now when it is time to rejoice.

> "Come then, my love,
> my lovely one, come.
> For see, winter is past,
> the rains are over and gone.
> The flowers appear on the earth.
> The season of glad songs has come,
> the cooing of the turtledove is heard
> in our land."
> (Song of Sol. 2:10-12)

The sun is sitting contentedly on our front steps. It looks as though he will be there for a while. I will take Joseph for a walk.

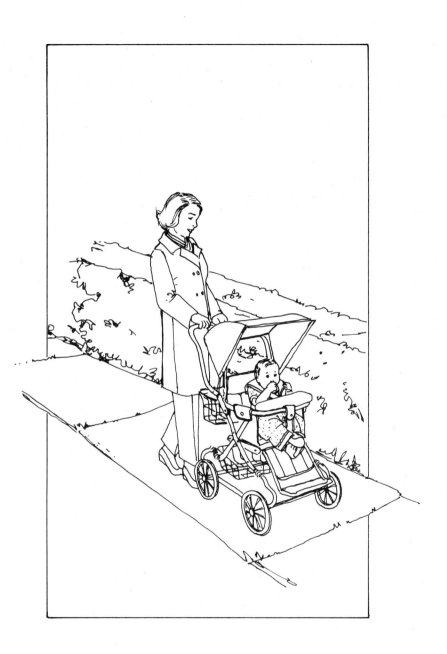